Transforming Healthcare with DevOps

A practical DevOps4Care guide to embracing the complexity of digital transformation

Jeroen Mulder

Henry Mulder

<packt>

BIRMINGHAM—MUMBAI

Transforming Healthcare with DevOps

Group Product Manager: Rahul Nair

Publishing Product Manager: Niranjan Naikwadi

Senior Editor: Romy Dias

Technical Editor: Rajat Sharma

Copy Editor: Safis Editing

Project Coordinator: Ashwin Dinesh Kharwa

Proofreader: Safis Editing

Indexer: Tejal Daruwale Soni

Production Designer: Prashant Ghare

Marketing Coordinator: Nimisha Dua

First published: November 2022

Production reference: 1041122

Published by Packt Publishing Ltd.

Livery Place

35 Livery Street

Birmingham

B3 2PB, UK.

ISBN 978-1-80181-731-8

www.packt.com

To everyone working in healthcare, all over the world. We owe you.

– Jeroen Mulder

To the doctors, nurses, public health officials, social workers, and first responders who are protecting us from COVID-19 and guarding our health.

– Henry Mulder

Contributors

About the authors

Jeroen Mulder (born 1970) is a principal business consultant and enterprise architect with the Japanese IT services company Fujitsu and a former principal cloud architect for Philips Precision Diagnosis. He's also a member of the city council of Emmen (the Netherlands) – the city where he was born and raised and still lives – with healthcare as a topic of special interest. Jeroen has previously written books about multi-cloud and DevOps for Packt Publishing.

I want to thank my wife, Judith, and my daughters, Rosalie and Noa, my precious family, for granting me all the space and support to spend so many hours writing – I realize that I need to seriously compensate for this time. A big thank you goes to Fujitsu, who allowed me to return to the Mothership. Lastly, I also want to thank the team at Packt for their faith and patience – especially Romy Dias, who did most of the editing once again – and for supporting us throughout this amazing journey.

Henry Mulder is a program manager for innovation with Trajectum, a care provider for intellectually disabled people needing guidance to participate safely in society, and a senior consultant at Q-Consult Zorg, a consultancy firm focused on practical change and transformations in healthcare.

He recently finished an assignment as a strategic advisor for MedMij, an interoperability governance foundation commissioned by the administrative collaboration between healthcare insurance companies and the Dutch Ministry of Health, Welfare and Sport, and a member of the NEN, the national committee on standards for health information systems.

First, my thanks to my partner, Maria, daughter, Larissa, and dog, Yara, for supporting me in writing this book. My gratitude to my colleagues at Q-Consult Zorg for being a great workplace that actively transforms healthcare for many care providers.

The communities of systems engineers (INCOSE) and system innovators (Si), for their discussions on what matters in transformation. Special thanks to the reviewers, Ray Deiotte and Gerrit Muller, for guiding us in the writing process. Finally, I want to thank all who have enlightened me with their insights.

About the reviewers

Raymond Deiotte has spent his career applying systems engineering theory and practice to the discipline of data exploitation across multiple industries. For nearly 20 years, he drove advanced decision-making automation with the application of systems of systems engineering principles and defined a taxonomy and modeling methodology to anticipate performance and behavior in the complex systems of systems. For the past 5 years, Raymond has brought those same concepts, techniques, and methodologies to US healthcare – redefining data governance, interoperability, and exploitation for clinicians and operators alike.

Gerrit Muller worked from 1980 until 1999 in the industry at Philips Healthcare and ASML. Since 1999, he has worked in research at Philips Research, the Embedded Systems Institute, and TNO in Eindhoven. He received his doctorate in 2004. In January 2008, he became a full professor of systems engineering at the **University of South-Eastern Norway** (**USN**) in Kongsberg, Norway. He continues to work at TNO in a part-time position. Since 2020, he is an INCOSE Fellow and Excellent Educator at USN.

Table of Contents

3

Unfolding the Complexity of Transformation   47

4

Including the Human Factor in Transformation   67

Part 2: Understanding and Working with Shared Mental Models

8

Learning How Interaction Works in Technology-Enabled Care Teams   147

9

Working with Complex (System of) Systems   163

Part 3: Applying TISH – Architecting for Transformation in Sustainable Healthcare

10

Assessments with TiSH   185

11

Planning, Designing, and Architecting the Transformation   203

12

Executing the Transformation   223

Preface

The topic of transforming healthcare is not new. As early as 2014, a report to the US President was issued with the following six recommendations:

- Accelerate alignment of payment systems with desired outcomes

- Increase access to relevant health data and analytics

- Provide technical assistance in systems engineering approaches

- Involve communities in improving healthcare delivery

- Share lessons learned from successful improvement efforts

- Train healthcare professionals in new skills and approaches

(Refer to *BETTER HEALTH CARE AND LOWER COSTS: ACCELERATING IMPROVEMENT THROUGH SYSTEMS ENGINEERING*.)

Although COVID-19 has put things in motion, it is still, as the World Health Organization puts it in various publications (refer to who.int), the technology to improve the health of populations that remains largely untapped, and there is immense scope for the use of digital health solutions.

Technology is an important driver for change, but in essence, we should design and plan for personalized health and not focus on just the technology. Healthcare transformation requires more than just technology: medical staff, supporting staff, and patients including their community such as next of kin, need to embrace it. We need a methodology to bring it all together – people, organizations, and technology – by creating a common understanding.

This book presents ways to build an understanding between stakeholders and agree jointly on the way forward. The intention of this book is to make developers aware of the models to understand the complexity of healthcare so they can recognize this complexity when involved in large healthcare transformation projects. We only briefly explain what each model is about. In the *Further reading* section at the end of each chapter, we refer to in-depth sources.

Every chapter of this book has a specific theme, providing a comprehensive overview of the challenges, the opportunities, and the approaches to deal with them in architecture and transformation. By the end of this book, you will be able to guide the digital transformation of global healthcare. The book discusses the impact of new technologies but addresses primarily a methodology or framework for common understanding in the first place. The framework is referred to as **Transformation in Sustainable Healthcare** (**TiSH**). In addition, you will also apply **Observe, Orient, Decide, Act** (**OODA**) principles and DevOps4Care to real-world examples, step by step.

By the end of this book, you will not only understand the issues and challenges of transformation of healthcare but also possess a workable, actionable solution in the form of a roadmap.

Who this book is for

This book is written for all interested in designing, building, and providing data-driven healthcare, specifically architects, consultants, engineers, and especially healthcare practitioners who want to embrace the complexity of the digital transformation of healthcare. The book will also be interesting for digital leaders, including C-level executives. Last but not least, this book is for anyone who is on a learning path to understand the world of technological innovation combined with healthcare and wants to be a part of it.

What this book covers

Chapter 1, *Understanding (the Need for) Transformation*, provides a broad introduction to the book, exploring the various challenges that healthcare faces, such as an aging population and scarcity of skilled staff.

Chapter 2, *Exploring Relevant Technologies for Healthcare*, explores the combined possibilities of new technologies, but always from the health experience perspective.

Chapter 3, *Unfolding the Complexity of Transformation*, is where we learn about the policies and regulations that form guardrails in healthcare and how this affects the transformation.

Chapter 4, *Including the Human Factor in Transformation*, is where we learn how to prevent humans – patients and care workers – from getting lost in regulations, systems, technology, and data. We must find a balance between man and machine.

Chapter 5, *Leveraging TiSH as Toolkit for Common Understanding*, provides an introduction to TiSH and DevOps4Care, including the underlying models and methods.

Chapter 6, *Applying the Panarchy Principle*, is about community building using ecocycles to overcome inhibitions and start planning the actual transformation.

Chapter 7, *Creating New Platforms with OODA*, introduces and teaches you how to work with the OODA loop as a way to drive the transformation using feedback loops.

Chapter 8, Learning How Interaction Works in Technology-Enabled Care Teams, introduces the **Journey Interaction Matrix (JIM)**, where we can follow the teams and monitor the activities throughout the health journey and interact with other teams in the ecosystem.

Chapter 9, Working with Complex (System of) Systems, is where we learn how to create a common understanding of how to integrate and transform into personal directed healthcare with the relevant solutions and systems, tread by tread in TiSH.

Chapter 10, Assessments with TiSH, is where we learn to perform assessments in healthcare, all in preparation for the transformation. For this, maturity models are introduced.

Chapter 11, Planning, Designing, and Architecting the Transformation, is where we put it all together, the concepts of TiSH and JIM, working with OODA loops, and forming the teams, and really start executing the transformation.

Chapter 12, Executing the Transformation, includes real-world examples of companies that have gone through a transformation. It ends with a big invitation to join the digital transformation of healthcare and help shape the future.

To get the most out of this book

Depending on your background prior to reading this book, we recommend you familiarize yourself with some concepts on which this book builds, such as the following:

- Peter Senge's *The Fifth Discipline* on systems thinking and the iceberg model

- Architectural reasoning from one of the reviewers of this book, Gerrit Muller

- *Enterprise DevOps for Architects*, by one of the authors of this book, Jeroen Mulder, published by Packt Publishing

- WHO's view on digital health: `https://www.who.int/health-topics/digital-health#tab=tab_1`

Download the color images

We also provide a PDF file that has color images of the screenshots and diagrams used in this book. You can download it here: `https://packt.link/2JSK8`.

Conventions used

> **Tips or important notes**
> Appear like this.

Get in touch

Feedback from our readers is always welcome.

General feedback: If you have questions about any aspect of this book, email us at `customercare@packtpub.com` and mention the book title in the subject of your message.

Errata: Although we have taken every care to ensure the accuracy of our content, mistakes do happen. If you have found a mistake in this book, we would be grateful if you would report this to us. Please visit `www.packtpub.com/support/errata` and fill in the form.

Piracy: If you come across any illegal copies of our works in any form on the internet, we would be grateful if you would provide us with the location address or website name. Please contact us at `copyright@packt.com` with a link to the material.

If you are interested in becoming an author: If there is a topic that you have expertise in and you are interested in either writing or contributing to a book, or a body of knowledge for a learning path please visit `authors.packtpub.com`.

Share your thoughts

Once you've read *Transforming Healthcare with DevOps*, we'd love to hear your thoughts! Scan the QR code below to go straight to the Amazon review page for this book and share your feedback.

`https://packt.link/r/1801817316`

Your review is important to us and the tech community and will help us make sure we're delivering excellent quality content.

Download a free PDF copy of this book

Thanks for purchasing this book!

Do you like to read on the go but are unable to carry your print books everywhere? Is your eBook purchase not compatible with the device of your choice?

Don't worry, now with every Packt book you get a DRM-free PDF version of that book at no cost.

Read anywhere, any place, on any device. Search, copy, and paste code from your favorite technical books directly into your application.

The perks don't stop there, you can get exclusive access to discounts, newsletters, and great free content in your inbox daily

Follow these simple steps to get the benefits:

1. Scan the QR code or visit the link below

https://packt.link/free-ebook/9781801817318

2. Submit your proof of purchase
3. That's it! We'll send your free PDF and other benefits to your email directly

Part 1:
Introducing Digital Transformation in Healthcare

After reading this part, you will have a good understanding of the transformation challenges and opportunities in healthcare. This part will introduce working with **Transformation in Sustainable Healthcare (TiSH)** as the reference framework for transformation. This part of the book is centered around a number of themes: urgency, possibilities, complexity, human measure, and TiSH itself.

The following chapters will be covered under this section:

- *Chapter 1, Understanding (the Need for) Transformation*
- *Chapter 2, Exploring Relevant Technologies for Healthcare*
- *Chapter 3, Unfolding the Complexity of Transformation*
- *Chapter 4, Including the Human Factor in Transformation*
- *Chapter 5, Leveraging TiSH as Toolkit for Common Understanding*

Understanding (the Need for) Transformation

While growing up, when things got tough, most of us ran to our mom for help and understanding. Well, as transforming healthcare can be very complicated indeed, we're also calling for our **MoM**, our **Model of Models**. She is called **TiSH**. We will introduce her first thing in this chapter.

Throughout this book, we remind you at the start of each chapter that MoM TiSH is always right behind you to get things in perspective.

The theme of this chapter is to set the stage for the transformation of healthcare into a far more real-time data-driven model. Why is this needed? What does it mean? How can we transform healthcare into this? And who do we involve for success?

This first chapter is a broad introduction to the book, exploring the various challenges that healthcare faces, such as an aging population and the scarcity of skilled staff. More people, with more and more treatable diseases, give an ever upward exponential trend of healthcare demand. We will learn about these challenges, how we can define the transformation with different stakeholders in the healthcare community, and who to involve to shape and drive this transformation. The most important lesson that we will learn is that it's all about the patient and the well-being of humans.

In this chapter, we're going to cover the following main topics:

- Setting the stage for transformation
- The urgency for transformation
- Understanding the role of diagnostics and observation
- Understanding the outcome on health and lifestyle
- Exploring the disciplines for common understanding

Setting the stage for transformation

For reasons we will dive into later, we want to transform healthcare, so we need to form a team or community with the required skills and experience to embrace this topic. We want to get our heads around it.

Looking for digital changes and innovation in healthcare can be a daunting task, let alone a whole digital transformation. It's a complex world that makes it hard to know where to begin and what to expect during a given time. We must embrace this complex world, whether we are from a medical, social, technical, consulting, or managerial discipline, and seek actionable ways to make the transformation happen.

We have to set the stage for the transformation team or community in which we will be playing our parts: on the supply side for care professionals, teams, and organizations to provision all kinds of healthcare, and on the demand side, the persons receiving treatments for their health and ever-increasing lifestyle improvements, so that they can participate in society.

Exploring this complexity, getting a common understanding across the disciplines, and knowing where to begin and how to proceed is the purpose of **Transformation into Sustainable Healthcare (TiSH)**.

For starters, and because this model will reappear in almost every chapter, we will introduce TiSH as an acronym, name, and model. The acronym is clear, the name is to make it personal and keep everything on a human level, and the model represents a placeholder for complexity, as demonstrated in this first figure:

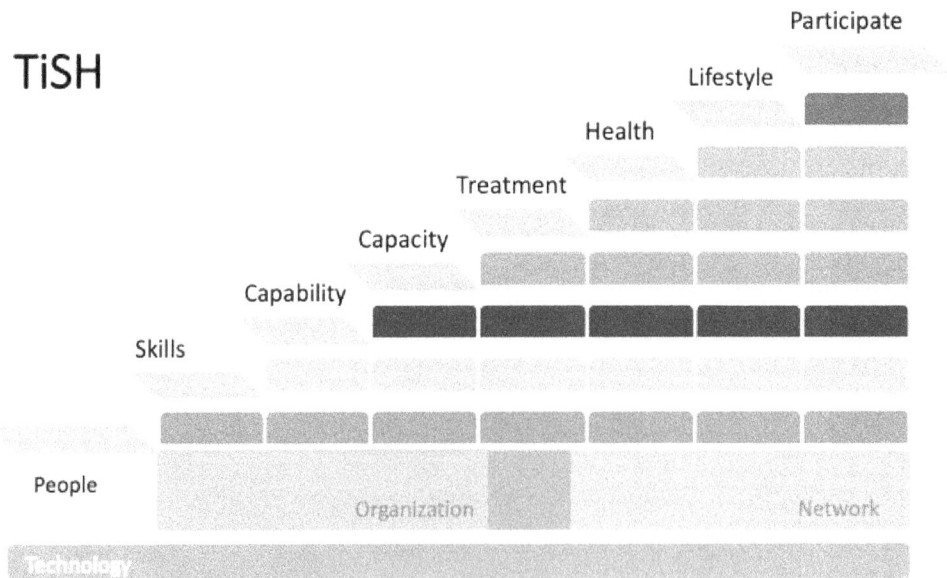

Figure 1.1 – The TiSH staircase for digital transformation in seven treads

The transformation objects at the foundation are **People** and **Technology**. The transformation itself is performed, tread by tread, as follows:

1. Learning digital **Skills** by individuals

2. Enabling the **Capabilities** of teams with technology

3. Ensuring enough **Capacity** for teams and their technology enablers

4. Providing quality data-driven **Treatments** to patients

5. Resulting in better-observed **Health**

6. Prevention via a healthier **Lifestyle**

7. The best outlook to **Participate** in society's activities

The lower four treads refer to the care provider's organization to deliver treatments, and the upper four treads are about the patient and their care network to work on their **Health** and **Lifestyle** and be able to **Participate**.

Note that each of these treads is already happening right now in some form without much technology, standardized work, or processing. In this book, we will discuss how to improve each tread with digital transformation and accelerate the move to the highest tread in a sustainable way. Here, we mean sustainable as in the use of human, technological, and environmental resources.

Our approach is to build the digital transformation, tread by tread, by doing the right things, in the right order, and at the right pace. In other words, the right systematic approach. With this, you can ask questions regarding which tread we stand on today, which treads are our objectives in the short, medium, and long term, and what we have to do to reach the new tread. Each time, a higher tread is built on the lower treads, putting the new tread on top. It's like building a staircase with pallets as building blocks, as represented in *Figure 1.1*, or rectangles with rounded upper corners. What these building blocks consist of will be revealed in the coming chapters.

The TiSH staircase forms a frame of mind to model the complexity of the transformation as a scaffold to fit knowledge, such as models and methods, into the transformation. In a way, it's used to build a model of models for the digital transformation of healthcare.

But first, let's start with the question of why? Why digital transformation, and why modeling?

Digital transformation is needed because of demographic, medical, technological, and especially digital advancements. We will explain the urgency of it in more detail later, where we will discuss what developments are driving these developments. Common or cross-disciplinary understanding is needed, as was already put forward in 1990 by Peter Senge in *The Fifth Discipline*. Here, systems thinking is the driving force realized through the shared modeling of complex developments, with a lot of disciplines working together.

In particular, it involves an combined understanding of the pillars of developing technology, business enabling, and providing care – in short, **Technology**, **Enabling**, and **Care**, as demonstrated in *Figure 1.2*:

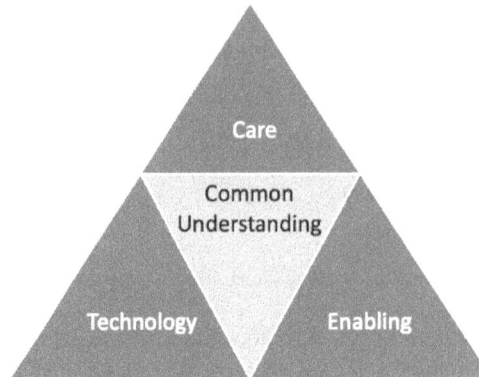

Figure 1.2 – Common understanding between technology, enabling, and care

For this understanding, generic and cross-disciplinary models can be used. We have to look for the **Goldilocks zone** of models for this cross-disciplinary understanding:

- Metaphors are too generic but suit initial recognition
- Single disciplinary models from their respective bodies of knowledge are too specific but are needed to detail and specify solutions
- Just right are generic models with some similarity with specialized models to be used in bridging these specialized models from two or more different disciplines

This book is our contribution to describing this fabric of understanding in such a way that the reader gets a foundation and toolbox for the journey of embracing the complexity of the digital transformation of healthcare. With this contribution, we invite all disciplines to join the transformation and secure enough transformation agents and resources to make it happen on the scale required.

We started our common understanding by using metaphors such as staircases and pallets as building blocks to build a sound foundation. These metaphors are very generic with no further explanation needed. However, having a common understanding is a bit more complex, as demonstrated in the tale of the village of blind people who encounter an elephant and try to describe it. Metaphors can be easily searched on the web. If you want to know more about these metaphors, you can look for them yourself in your further reading. Try searching for the phrase "elephant metaphor."

Additionally, cross-disciplinary generic models can be found relatively easily on the internet, as they are widely accepted by many disciplines. We will discuss how to apply them to the digital transformation process, referring to other sources for more information and further reading on the model itself or other usages.

Also, we will use some specific models to be able to bind the disciplinary bodies of knowledge. These will be explained in more detail as they form the main threads of reasoning and exploration to design jointly transformational solutions. By combining models, we get new insights to reason about and explore these solutions. Also, it helps to translate from one viewpoint or discipline to another, helping the process of common understanding.

Digital twins

Next to this modeling for common understanding of healthcare, it is useful to build a digital twin, a real-time virtual representation of real-world entities, activities, and processes. We can distinguish three of these digital twins:

- The digital landscape itself

- The medical and social processes

- The avatar of a person

Let's talk about the avatar, which is a digital representation of the patient. We will follow the avatar as we go through the different stages of transforming healthcare. The avatar will help us in understanding what's in it for the patient. We cannot predict the future, but we do think that we will have a digital twin of ourselves soon: an avatar that holds all the data about our health (known as a quantified self) and tells our doctors what they need to know, a simulation of a person for clinical diagnostics based on input from, for example, scans, examinations, and medication.

This will help a clinician set precise diagnostics and define precise interventions without heavily impacting the patient. The avatar will help them to stay focused on the patient. And that's what this book is all about: the patient or, even better, how to prevent an individual from ever becoming one.

With modeling, you can specify and quantify the healthcare in all aspects so that simulations can be designed to explore different scenarios of the transformation. Based on this, better solutions can be made.

We hope these digital twins will create feedback loops to self-direct the actions to the desired state of common understanding, sustainability, and health.

The urgency for transformation

The first big question we ask is why a digital transformation is needed. So, before we get to the transformation and the selection of methodologies themselves and plan the transformation, first, we need to understand why we (urgently) need the transformation and what drives this transformation.

In all the rapid advancements and increasingly overwhelming scientific and technological progress, we tend to forget that, at end of the day, it's all about humans. So, what is in it for you personally, whatever your role is? That is the question we asked ourselves when we started writing this book. From our professional roles in healthcare technology, as a patient or the next of kin of a patient, and as members of society, it's the human factor that really counts. Therefore, this book will be 100 percent person- or people-centric, meaning that we will look at healthcare from the patient's and caregiver's perspectives the entire time. This is our perspective for the following assessments and quest for understanding.

On one hand, we see many great opportunities in things such as big data, machine learning, and artificial intelligence in combination with bioengineering. However, we also see the potential undesired effect on people and society. We, as people and as a society, need time to digest the new possibilities before taking well-founded decisions. The consequences can be profound.

With that in mind, first, we must put a stake in the ground and understand what drives the urgency for changing healthcare. This urgency is mainly caused by demographic drivers and disruptive economic drivers.

Understanding demographic drivers

Although certainly not complete, we will give some examples in which to understand demographic drivers:

- One obvious driver is aging: we are getting older. That fact alone is already driving demand for care, in both emerging and developed economies. Figures from the United Nations show an increase in the global population by 1 billion people in 2025. That's only 3 years from when this book was written. Of that 1 billion extra people, around 300 million will have reached the age of 65 or more.

- But there are more demographic factors that we need to consider. For instance, there will significant growth of the so-called middle class due to developments within countries. So, how's that a driver for healthcare? The middle class will have greater and better access to a more *luxurious* lifestyle, which might lead to the occurrence of more obesity and other health problems that will burden the healthcare system.

- Growth is not equally divided across the planet. It's expected that the population on the African continent will double by 2050, while the population in Europe will shrink.

- There's a downside to the preceding point. With the growth of developing countries, there's another trend that is becoming visible: the **World Health Organization** (**WHO**) calculated that, in 1990, breast cancer, diabetes, stroke, and other **noncommunicable diseases** (**NCDs**) formed 25 percent of the total amount of death and chronic illnesses in these countries. That number will rise to 80 percent by 2040 in some of the economically rising countries.

- Where people would likely die a century ago because of a certain disease that could not be treated, we are now able to cure a lot of these diseases due to immense scientific progress.

Cancer is probably the best example here. Although it's still life-threatening, a good number of cancers can now be treated with the prospect of good outcomes for the patient. Again, the issue is that access to cures and treatments is not evenly divided across the globe.

- Finally, a very important driver is the scarcity of staff in care. This is a global issue. In some countries, it has been calculated that, over the coming years, one-third of all jobs will be in healthcare, something that has been accelerated by the COVID-19 pandemic. This is not a sustainable model. To make it slightly worse, in some countries, care institutions are recruiting staff in other countries that need skilled personnel just as urgently as anywhere else, causing a "brain drain" in some parts of the world and enlarging the inequality of access to care.

The net result of all of this is that people will need complex, coordinated care for a longer period. There will be more people to take care of, and these people will live longer because we also have the capabilities to cure more diseases. On the other hand, there's a huge risk that we can't deliver that care because we don't have the skilled staff to do so. This is causing the urgency to transform healthcare into a more sustainable model – a model that also allows us to scale it across the globe.

Understanding disruption in healthcare

Healthcare is already transforming, as we will discover in this section. Disruption is happening, as in almost any other industry, by highly innovative newcomers on the market. Global initiatives have been launched, disrupting traditional healthcare. We see non-healthcare industries expanding into this new market. This includes retail, wellness, and even telecom companies. They all have good business reasons for expanding into this market: healthcare is growing in the global market with tremendous opportunities. From a commercial perspective, healthcare is becoming a more and more attractive space to be in as a business.

On the other hand, we have no choice because of the increasing demand that traditional players can't address sufficiently anymore. New entrants are leaping into the gap. It's inevitable: a collaboration between the traditional stakeholders and new, private, commercial initiatives is required to meet the expectations of patients and clients. These patients and clients are getting used to on-demand and fast service, with the continuous improvement of products and services alongside comfort and convenience experienced with the likes of Uber, Booking.com, and other platforms. Healthcare is like any consumer market, acting with the same principles as, for instance, retail. The consumer sets the pace of innovation: on demand, ease of access, ease of use, reliability, always on, anytime, anywhere, and anyplace. This comes with a huge shift in the way healthcare must reshape its delivery model and become more agile.

At the same time, we need to control costs, so solutions need to be cost-effective. A shift to more prevention, on one hand, and more at-home care, on the other hand, are the North Stars here. Promoting wellness, a healthy lifestyle, and preventing diseases should, in the first place, benefit people and, at the same time, drive costs down – a very attractive perspective for payers and governments. Plus, the solutions are cost-effective when they are scalable. These solutions are developed once and deployed many times, preferably on a global scale.

Understanding the business context

The big change is the shift to prevention through lifestyle and behavior rather than cure. The WHO and many national government institutions have highlighted this more and more on their agenda. The COVID-19 measures on social distancing are a good example.

Therefore, a lot of new companies in healthcare are focusing on prevention by stimulating a healthy lifestyle. This is a global trend where we start to acknowledge that healthcare doesn't start in the office of a doctor but in our personal lives and the way we take care of ourselves, for instance, with our lifestyle choices.

A well-known example is the various wearables that track movements – they monitor basic parameters such as your heart rate, sleep score, and activity points, and based on that data, provide advice for exercising. Some of these devices – think of the Apple Watch – already go the extra mile and make it possible to produce **electrocardiograms** (**ECGs**). Other apps measure an individual's body fat percentage by using the camera on their smartphone – one of the features of the Halo View by Amazon.

Devices such as wearables and apps simply help people to maintain a healthy lifestyle. We probably all know what's good for us and what's not. Health is impacted by lifestyle:

- Inactivity
- Unhealthy diets
- Too much alcohol
- Smoking
- Not enough sleep
- Too much stress

We know all of this, but apparently, it helps if someone or something helps keep us to stay alert to these factors. The biggest alert that a person could get is a serious health issue that results from an unhealthy lifestyle. Therefore, lifestyle is a very important driver in overall healthcare architecture and the transformation to more sustainable healthcare.

A sense of urgency is about pace – the pace of change. Many industries already adopted this new paradigm some time ago and started changing their business models for mainly one reason: they were forced to because of disrupting models that had been introduced into their markets.

Famous examples include Uber, which disrupted the market for taxis, and Airbnb, which did the same with traditional leisure. Are we seeing this in healthcare, too? The short answer is yes. There's a shift happening already. In this book, we will look at some of these disrupting initiatives, for example, Amazon Care and a famous Dutch initiative called Buurtzorg that has gone international. The message of Buurtzorg is to *simplify the systems and start again from the patient perspective*.

> **Tip**
>
> Although Buurtzorg started as a Dutch initiative, the model is marketed internationally. We will refer to Buurtzorg a few times in this book, but more information can also be found at `https://www.buurtzorg.com/about-us/`.

Healthcare made easy, says the website of Amazon Care, promising care when the patient wants it, in the way they want it, and at the time they want it, fully focusing on the health experience. It should not be a surprise that Amazon brought this to the market. It's derived from the guiding principle on which Jeff Bezos started Amazon: the company and its employees are obsessed with the customers of Amazon. Amazon calls this *customer obsessed*. In the case of Amazon Care, this becomes *patient obsessed*, including *quality time with your team of doctors and nurse practitioners – on demand*.

One other factor that makes Amazon Care and Buurtzorg great examples for this book to study is that both concepts are fully scalable and work according to agile principles. In *Chapter 8*, *Learning How Interaction Works in Technology-Enabled Care Teams*, we will learn more about these principles.

> **Note**
>
> A number of books have been written explaining the development and management philosophy of Amazon. Recent books include comprehensive descriptions of the *working backward* methodology that Amazon uses to create new services and products. This method was also used in creating Amazon Care: starting with the patient or the client, and their need, and then working backward to solutions that would address this. It's a fundamentally different methodology of doing architecture. Although we will use Amazon Care as an example in this book, we will not go into detail about *working backward*.

The question is how to determine what must be done for health, when, and where. This is where diagnostics come in. Let's get some insights into that in the next section.

Understanding the role of diagnostics and observation

The Mayo Clinic in the United States is perceived to be a lighthouse in modern healthcare, although the clinic was already founded back in the late 19th century. The American-based clinic puts tremendous effort into getting diagnostics right from the very first moment, for a lot of different reasons.

In the book *Management Lessons from Mayo Clinic*, founder Dr. William Mayo (1895) says: *Above all things let me urge upon you the absolute necessity of careful examinations for the purpose of diagnosis. My own experience has been that the public will forgive you an error in treatment more readily than one in diagnosis, and I fully believe that more than one-half of the failures in diagnosis are due to hasty or unmethodical examinations.*

Dr. Mayo figured out that an inaccurate or even wrong diagnosis would cause serious further problems to a patient and the quality of care.

Diagnostics have a decisive impact on the quality of care and patient safety by highlighting the following:

- Disease prevention through early screening

- Discovery of any diseases at an early stage through the accurate diagnosis of early symptoms

- Prognosis of the course of the disease, including determining the effectiveness of treatments and medications such as antibiotics

- Decisions on follow-up treatments and monitoring the long-term effectiveness of those treatments

Diagnostics is aiming for improving patient care. Getting an accurate diagnosis is crucial. Getting an accurate diagnosis in a timely matter is even more crucial. Healthcare institutions are investing heavily in diagnostics. Let's take the aforementioned Mayo Clinic as an example.

In April 2021, the clinic announced massive investments in a new platform to deliver AI-driven clinical decision support through remote monitoring. It cooperates with other companies that develop algorithms for the early detection of diseases and collect data from remote devices to support clinical decisions. These two companies – Anumana and Lucem Health – are both start-ups. This is what we will see in the future: *traditional* healthcare players seeking cooperation with start-ups that deliver cutting-edge technology to enhance care.

Mayo Clinic's Platform President, Dr. John Halamka, is convinced that the upcoming technology in AI and data science will result in a breakthrough in disease detection and, with that, a better perspective for patients. However, in the statement, he added that this is not just about technology – he also stressed the importance of patient engagement and cultural changes in healthcare to make it happen (source: Healthcare IT News, April 2021).

So, diagnostics is important, but how is it driving transformation in healthcare? Getting better, faster results from diagnostics can save impactful interventions, long-term treatments, and more speedy recovery. Again, we need to keep the patient as the focus. Less impactful interventions, less need for long-term treatments, and speedy recoveries will, in the first place, benefit the patient. And, as a more than welcome side effect, it will drive the costs for healthcare down – at least that's what economic specialists in the field expect.

With that, we are entering the field of precision diagnostics and precision medicine. A number of studies have been executed to show the cost-effectiveness of precision diagnosis and precision medicine. Precision diagnosis and precision medicine are decisive in the following ways:

- Reducing the risk of treatment by trial and error

- Reducing the risk of over-prescription

- Shortening the time before treatment is started

- Decreasing the time that a patient has to spend in hospital or care institutions

The contradiction lies in the fact that precision diagnosis and precision medicine require substantial investments. However, studies from the University of Utah (source: `https://www.cms.gov/ Research-Statistics-Data-and-Systems/Statistics-Trends-and-Reports/ NationalHealthExpendData/NationalHealthAccountsHistorical`) show that these upfront investments can save expenditures in the long run when it comes to the execution of treatment. More importantly, the studies show that the quality of life of the patient is improving with accurate, precision diagnosis and precision medicine.

Going back to the previous section, we can see that people have already invested in smartwatches that observe their vital signs and give advice or alerts when needed. This observation and subsequent prefiltering allow for the early detection of possible health conditions but will also limit the influx of people for screening and diagnostics.

Understanding the outcome on health and lifestyle

There's one driver that will benefit a person's health even more, as we learned earlier, and that's lifestyle – that is, preventing an individual from becoming a patient. We will explain this using the *health experience* shortened as **HeX**, similarly to **UX** for **User eXperience** in the DevOps world. This HeX is the first reference model we will use to understand each other.

First, we need to explain what the **HeX** is. It refers to the health activities of a person, varying from participating in daily life to being treated and (chronically) nursed as a patient. We use *omniversal* care to represent the lifetime journey through which a person, as a patient, travels in terms of required care from the cradle to the grave.

> **Note**
> We are using the word **omniversal**: **omnidirectional** and **universal**. This applies to all health activities from every direction at the same time.

The following diagram shows the omniversal care in the HeXagon for health experience:

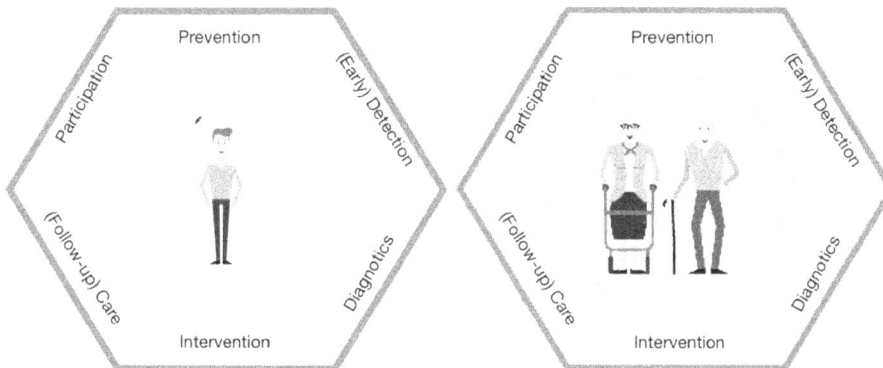

Figure 1.3 – Omniversal care HeXagon to represent the Health eXperience (HeX)

The basic model is firmly patient-centric, with the activities of the person as a reference. At any given time, the person is participating in the daily life of society, conducting – more or less – prevention activities such as sports or walking, and getting regular check-ups or tests such as for colon cancer. A patient will probably visit the **General Practitioner** (**GP**). If required, further medical diagnosis is performed along with treatment such as intervention with medication, exercises, or an operation. The patient might receive either short-term or chronic nursing care. This can be for one or more diseases (co-morbidity).

The goal of any person is, implicitly or explicitly, to stay active on the upper half of the hexagon: participation, prevention, and early detection. That has a direct relation with lifestyle. Over the past few decades, medical science concluded that a healthy lifestyle is preventing a lot of commonly known diseases. An unhealthy lifestyle can lead to obesity, which, in turn, can lead to all sorts of health issues such as diabetes, cardiovascular diseases, or orthopedic problems.

Let's get back to the demographic changes that have had an impact on global healthcare. In the first section, we discussed the rise of noncommunicable diseases in economically rising countries.

A study by Thomas J. Bollyky is a good example and reference for this topic. In his study, he relates the increase in cancers, diabetes, cardiovascular diseases, chronic respiratory illnesses, and other noncommunicable diseases in low-income countries to the *increased prevalence of key modifiable behavioral risks, such as unhealthy diets and tobacco use, and reductions in the infectious diseases that disproportionately kill children and adolescents.*

Worse still, these are also countries that are not well prepared to deal with these diseases because they hardly have any access to proper healthcare. However, again, it shows the major effect that lifestyle has on health.

> **Note**
> The full study, entitled *Lower-Income Countries That Face The Most Rapid Shift In Noncommunicable Disease Burden Are Also The Least Prepared*, is available at `https://www.healthaffairs.org/doi/full/10.1377/hlthaff.2017.0708`.

The examples of Buurtzorg and Amazon Care can also be depicted in the omniversal care hexagon. The first extension of the HeX shows the principle of Buurtzorg.

The HeXagon on the right-hand side of *Figure 1.3* shows how Buurtzorg is creating an inner supportive hexagon to avoid outer professional care, if possible, and rely on the local community.

Amazon Care is organizing the care ecosystem around the family of their employees to optimize participation, as shown in the following diagram:

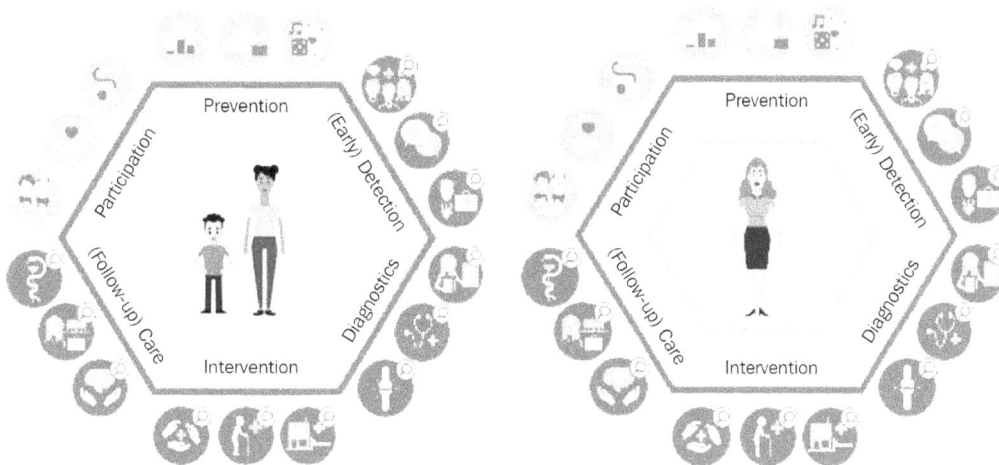

Figure 1.4 – HeXagon of health experience showing the care ecosystem

Combining the two leads to the complete Omniversal Care HeXagon representing the patient-centric care ecosystem of self, social, and medical care. The hexagon on the right-hand side shows the complete HeX, the hexagon for health experience. Support comes from the social (the yellow or light circles) providers and medical care from (the blue or dark circles) providers.

HeX is the representation of the complete individual healthcare ecosystem. Every citizen on earth should have such an ecosystem available. So, that's the stage on which we set our transformation challenge.

Exploring the disciplines for common understanding

We have set our challenge. Who do we need? Looking at Amazon, they utilize their platform to provide the care needed for their employees with the same rigor of customer obsession as with their logistics services.

A platform creates value by enabling interactions between two or more groups. In the case of healthcare, this is the providers, patients, and people who want to stay healthy. A platform has two major parts. One is the digital technology and the other is the community of involved people, care workers, and patients alike. Building a platform requires disciplines to build the technology and communities:

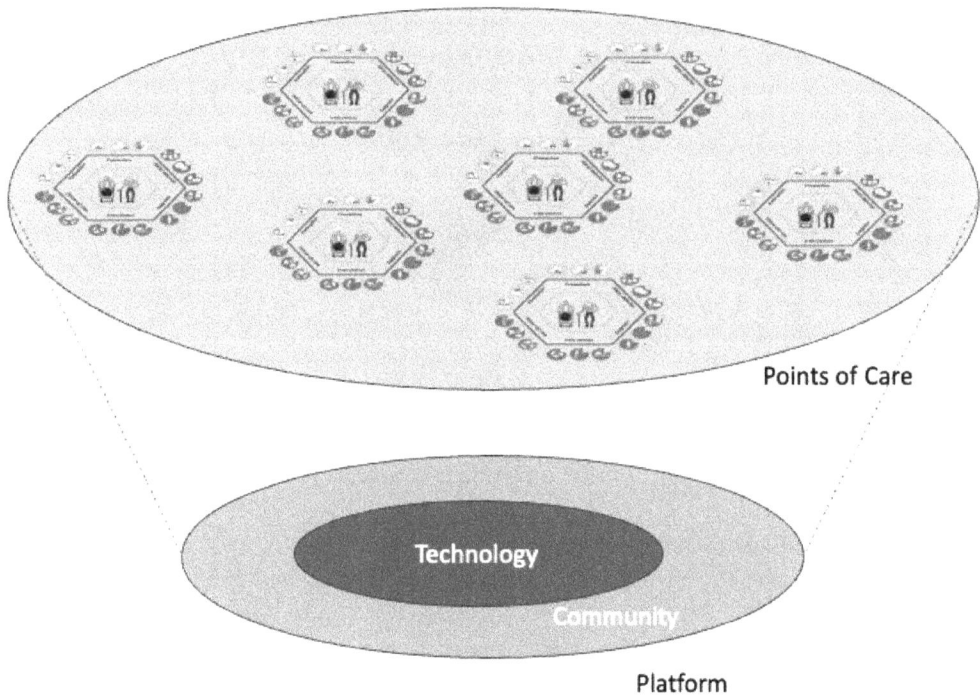

Figure 1.5 – The platform consists of technology and communities to serve at the point of care

The two disciplines that can build this are systems engineering with a technology approach for the platform and systems innovation for the community-building approach. So, how do we involve our transformation teams in these disciplines?

Working with system engineers on health

System engineers focus on how to design, integrate, and manage complex systems over their life cycles. For a successful transformation, we have to understand how they think and work, especially in their role as architects.

Getting to a model that supports HeX means that healthcare must adopt agile, highly scalable concepts and embrace **DevOps** as part of the transformation. It's a guided, agile way of developing solutions to execute this transformation. Applying this to healthcare transformation leads to something that we call **DevOps4Care**. This is where technology architects and consultants from medicine and healthcare enterprises closely work together to find the best solutions for the patient.

Ultimately, this book is about DevOps4Care: an agile way to create new, sustainable solutions in a speedy manner that will improve healthcare. It requires a complex transformation. In *Chapter 3, Unfolding the Complexity of Transformation*, we will discuss the complexity of this transformation in much more detail.

Understanding the difference between the architect and medical or business consultants requires a common reference such as we already introduced with metaphors and the book-related reference models of TiSH and HeX. In this section, we will further discuss these references and models.

Architects shape structures. They do not predict the future, although enterprise and business architects have visions of the future just as real estate architects do. What collectively binds us – or better yet, what we have in common – is that all architects and consultants come from a perspective where something is needed or desired. In business, that typically starts with business requirements, usually expressed by the consultant representing the many stakeholders. The business sees a demand, formulates requirements to address this demand, and sets these requirements as a starting point for creating architecture that, in the end, will result in a solution or a product. Healthcare isn't different from that general principle, the only difference is that we now have a lot of medical-oriented stakeholders.

As an architect, the architecture in healthcare also is derived from the medical and business perspective. It's the reason why all enterprise architecture models start with the business view. **The Open Group Architecture Framework** (**TOGAF**), the enterprise architecture method of The Open Group, is a good example and an industry standard for architecture. TOGAF starts reasoning from the business: what are the requirements of the business, which, in our case, is healthcare? But TOGAF is a technology perspective. We need to build an understanding of the healthcare enterprise and medicine itself.

Each person will have their own way of picturing and reasoning the transformation. We need to find a way in which to get a common understanding as it will take some effort. How do we understand each other in the following questions? Why do we need to transform healthcare, and why is it so urgent to do something about it? How do we define that something?

You will understand by reading, reasoning (even while reading this book), exploring your ideas together with the other stakeholders, integrating them within the constraints given by the qualities of the environment, and finally specifying it in such a way that others also can understand it to do their tasks in the transformation. We can make good use of *Architectural Reasoning* to achieve this common understanding.

> Tip
>
> To make this book a more effective read, we advise you to have a look at *Architectural Reasoning* by Gerrit Muller. A link is provided in the *Further reading* section.

The takeaway from *Architectural Reasoning* is that you mostly reason in your own mind, going back and forth on all aspects, viewpoints, and details. By telling stories and/or interacting with someone who is telling stories, together, you explore what possible solutions could be considered. In these stories, metaphors and generic models are used. They are used in the next step to formally integrate the insights within the constraints of budget, laws, and required qualities leading to the description (specification) of the actual solutions based on selected and jointly understood specific models.

A common understanding can be advanced by using reference models to which the different disciplines can relate equally. From the common understanding the various disciplines can agree on joint insights and understand the real needs behind the wishes and demands of patients. As we mentioned earlier for the transformation, we need perspectives on the following three pillars:

- Technology to be developed and led by the architect
- Enabling business operations and healthcare enterprises led by business consultants
- Care activities led by the respective medical disciplines

As a side note, together, the first characters of the above pillar form the acronym **Technology-Enabled Care (TEC)**. Remember this acronym for later.

These three perspectives are different. Let's find out more by giving each perspective some attention and learning about their differences.

Understanding the architecture of technology

As mentioned earlier, architects are familiar with TOGAF when they are designing digital systems. **Requirements** management sits in the middle of this. TOGAF recommends working with business scenarios as a technique to discover and document business requirements and, by doing that, drive the architecture. Now, how would that work in healthcare? The answer to that question is that it works exactly the same.

> **Tip**
>
> Another thing that might draw attention is the fact that architecture is not driven by technology. On the contrary, architecture is driven by business and that results in requirements for the technology that can be used as an enabler to achieve your business goals. In other words, it's never about technology in the first place.
>
> Read the last sentence a few times over, and reflect on it. It's an important point of departure in reasoning about and exploring the transformation.

In this book, we will look at the most important driver for doing architecture in healthcare: the needs of the patient. Our business objective is sustainable healthcare where we can take care of more people, improve their lives, and increase the quality of care. Where is the input for these requirements coming from? In the previous sections, we studied some of the most important drivers: demographic changes resulting in the aging of people and scarcity of staff, the impact of diagnostics resulting in more treatable diseases, and change in lifestyle. It's all causing increasing pressure on the need for sustainable healthcare.

The architect is responsible for the overall quality of the architecture. But creating architecture is not an isolated process. The architect has to work with different requirements, coming from various stakeholders that are mostly represented or advised by consultants. These stakeholders all have different needs, concerns, demands, wishes, and expectations. The architect will have to meet the stakeholders' views on what they perceive as a good outcome of architecture. Let's make that a bit more tangible.

The stakeholders in healthcare are the care providers, such as GPs, hospitals, clinicians, and care staff. Then, we have regulatory bodies such as governments setting regulations, rules, and laws for the delivery of care. Next, we have the institutions that pay for the care, typically insurance companies or public funds. Another stakeholder is the suppliers of services and goods, such as pharmaceutical companies and companies that deliver high-tech equipment to hospitals. And of course, the patient is likely the most important stakeholder. At the end of the day, it's all about their well-being.

Working with reference architecture to enable business operations

How do architects put all of this together: the requirements, the stakeholders' views, the objectives, and the architectural methods? How do architects address technology, healthcare enterprise, and healthcare itself in the architecture?

For development, we refer to **Agile** and DevOps as a reference. Let's concentrate on the healthcare enterprise enabling the operations of care activities.

Here, the reference architectures for healthcare might be of help. An example of such a reference architecture on the TOGAF side is the **Reference Architecture for Health (RA4H)** by Oliver-Matthias Kipf, as shown in the following diagram of health enterprise activities:

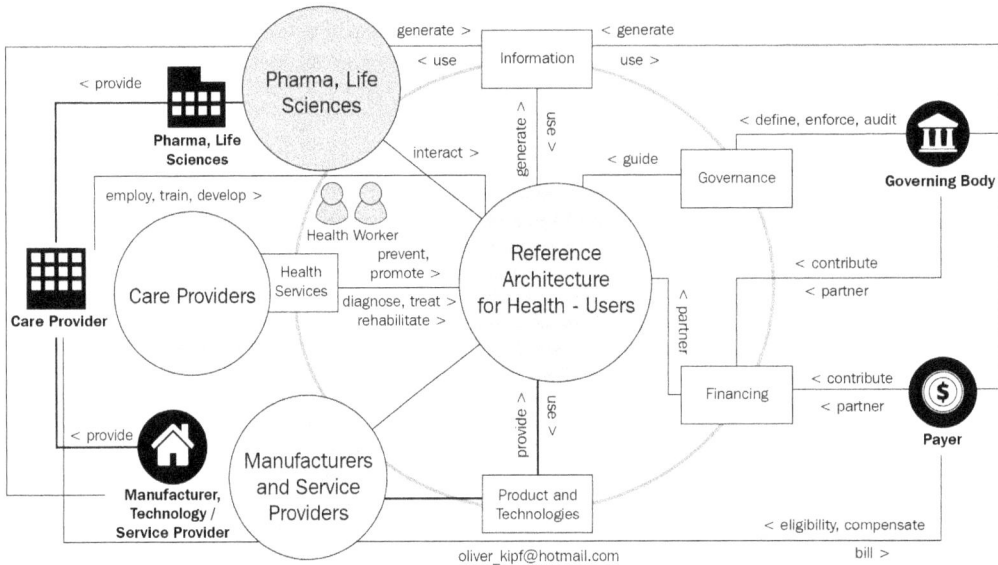

Figure 1.6 – Reference Architecture for Health (RA4H), used with the consent of O.M. Kipf

The key in this architecture is the position of the patient, who is the health user. The focus is on the personal health journey and how stakeholders in the ecosystem can provide services that ensure a better, healthier, and safer life for the patient. As Kipf rightfully explains, the ultimate aim of the architecture is to help improve healthcare, but from the health user's perspective.

The reference architecture shows how the ecosystem around the user is built, who the stakeholders are, and where the requirements originate from in terms of people, services, processes, products, and data. The architecture connects the domains of the stakeholders, collects the inputs along the patient's journey, and enables a structured way to get to the desired output – better health – as shown in the next diagram:

Required Input

- Health Workers
- Health Services and Care Processes
- Medicine, Devices, Consumer Products, Spare Parts
- Healthcare-Related Data

Along the journey and at every step

Personal Health Journey   2021   2022   2023

|Care Episode| | Care Episode | | Care Episode |

Desired Output

oliver_kipf@hotmail.com

- Better Health
- Meaningful Health Information

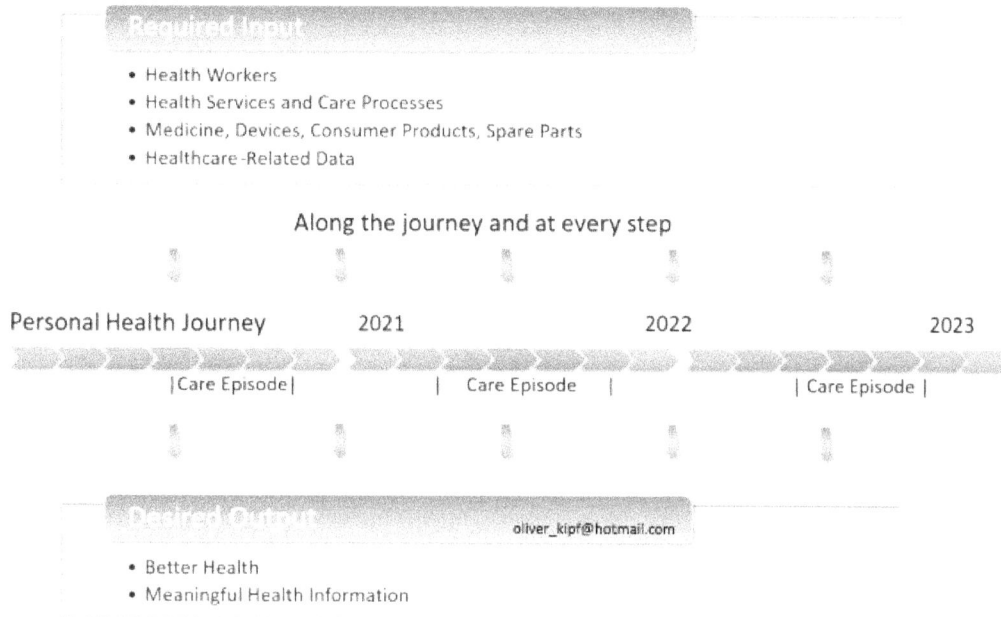

Figure 1.7 – The personal health journey, used with the consent of O.M. Kipf

Architecture is about setting goals and planning the transformation to achieve these goals. It's about building, delivering services, managing these services, and continuously improving these services, while also managing the risks that threaten to derail the transformation. That can't be done in isolation – you need all of the partners within the ecosystems to work together with a common understanding.

With such a reference model, it is possible to relate technological architecture with the business needs of the healthcare enterprise. But what about the care community?

Working with communities on medical outcomes

Also, for medical goals, we need a reference model, preferably omniversal with medical and social care combined if we want to have a successful transformation. There are many medical models out there, but for our purpose and to demonstrate getting a common understanding of the TEC pillars, we will show you how to relate to the care episodes of the personal health journey in *Figure 1.7*. Note that several care episodes can be in parallel and executed by different care providers, which have to be aligned in their desired output. These care providers form a community around the patient.

An example of such a reference model is **Integrated Care (INCA)**, as shown in the next diagram:

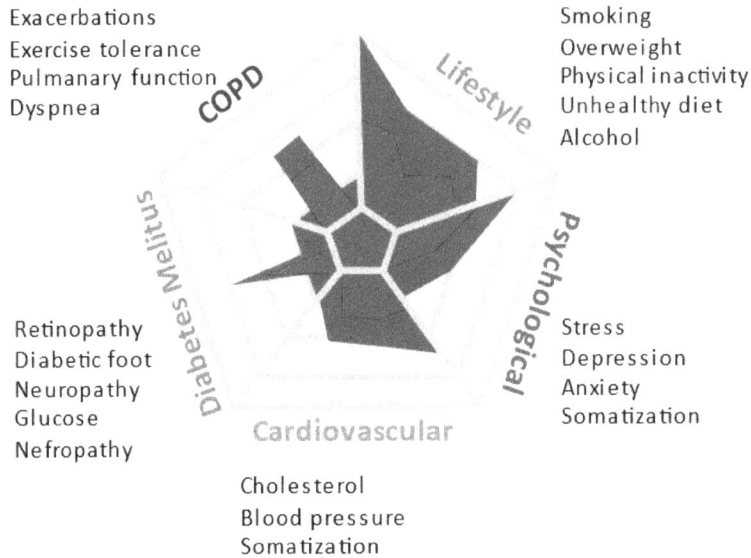

Figure 1.8 – Integrated Care (INCA) spider diagram, used with the consent of Dr. Javier Asin

The preceding example of an INCA spider diagram depicts five interdependent health conditions, each with its own care provider and care episodes. The medical and social professionals coordinate the interventions within these episodes for each condition to maximize the overall outcome for the patient, which is better health. In this case, an improvement over one year is shown in this spider diagram. The color red refers to this year, and the color blue refers to last year. A lower score means a lower care intensity in the episode. The care intensity is either self-care, social care, ambulatory medical care, or medical care in a GP practice or clinic. This spider is used to define the person's health journey in a patient-centric way by deciding which health condition is impacting their participation in society the most.

This spider method was successfully introduced in Suriname by Dr. Javier Asin. We will elaborate on this in *Chapter 9, Working with Complex (System of) Systems*, where we will talk about integration and integrated care that requires the building of a care community consisting of social and medical care.

In the next chapters, we will explore how to relate these three TEC pillars and get a common understanding between stakeholders on all levels.

The wicked challenge – thinking patient-centric

Patient-centric thinking adds much to the complexity and has to be addressed by the architecture, or otherwise, it leads either to chaos or excessive costs. Therefore, in this book, we will work with many reference architectures and models, all with the same goal: transforming healthcare to improve it for the patient from the perspective of the patient's own activities.

Finding and linking these reference models with each other for common understanding is what we will address in the coming chapters to build the health experience with HeX.

We will look at different methodologies such as **observe–orient–decide–act** (**OODA**), **Moment of Truth** (**MoT**), and **Ecosystem Micro Communities** (**EMC**) to form shared mental models that help us align viewpoints in transforming healthcare. *Chapter 7, Creating New Platforms with OODA*, will introduce a way of working in such an architecture, *Chapter 8, Learning How Interaction Works in Technology-Enabled Care Teams*, covers how to realize MoT in the health experience, and *Chapter 9, Working with Complex (System of) Systems,* discusses EMC.

We promised to be completely human-centric. The **Reference Architecture for Healthcare** (**RA4H**), which is derived from TOGAF principles, does just that: it focuses on the person, the patient, or the *health user.*

But we are also setting the scene for the digital transformation of healthcare, for all the reasons that we discussed in the previous sections. We need to transform to get to a more sustainable model for the delivery of healthcare. TiSH will help us in getting our heads around this wicked challenge.

In summary, healthcare transformation is about the following:

- Creating platform solutions that address comfort and convenience for the patient – 100% patient-centric for the outcome of a healthy lifestyle with a positive outlook on participation
- Creating platform solutions that are continuously improving the enabling business by adopting agile principles and community building
- Creating platform solutions that are cost-effective by adopting scalability as a driver to cover the world over
- Above all, creating a common understanding between technology, enabling, and care

So, where's the technology in all of this? Health technology can, and will, certainly enable the creation of sustainable solutions. In *Chapter 2, Exploring Relevant Technologies for Healthcare*, we will explore the innovations of technology in healthcare, but always with that one question in mind: what's in it for the patient?

Summary

This chapter was an introduction to this book. We set our challenge for the transformation. We introduced the TiSH staircase with the seven treads of transformation. We studied the various inputs that will drive the transformation of healthcare. We learned that drivers come from major global trends. Demographic trends such as the aging population and scarcity of skilled staff cause and increase the upward pressure on global healthcare systems. Next, we studied how precision diagnosis, precision medicine, and lifestyle are proven methods to drive costs of healthcare down and, at the same time, help to improve the quality of life of patients.

The most important lesson that we learned in this chapter is that the transformation of healthcare must be about the patient. This is something that requires a common understanding between all stakeholders and an understanding of TEC. In the final sections, we introduced the architecture of healthcare systems, using enterprise architecture methodologies such as TOGAF, the RA4H, and the community for INCA as a reference to digitization, medicine, and health itself. We can use these models to collect the jointly understood requirements for changing healthcare, but always with the patient as the center of the architectural and community models that we use.

In this chapter, we also introduced HeX: the healthcare experience, showing how care really can be organized from the patient's perspective, with scalable, even disruptive solutions. It forms a further introduction to this book in which we will study new models and agile ways of working to transform healthcare into a more sustainable system. It forms the introduction to DevOps4Care.

In the next chapter, we will explore the major emerging technology trends in healthcare.

Further reading

- *The Fifth Discipline, the art and practice of the learning organization*, Peter M. Senge, 1990, Crown Publishing Group.

- *Architectural Reasoning Explained*, Gerrit Muller, University of South-Eastern Norway-NISE: `https://www.gaudisite.nl/ArchitecturalReasoningBook.pdf`.

- *Management Lessons from Mayo Clinic* by Leonard L. Berry and Kent. D. Seltman, 2008, McGraw-Hill.

- Oliver Matthias Kipf, 2020, The Open Group blog: `https://blog.opengroup.org/2020/12/29/reference-architecture-for-healthcare-ra4h-core-capabilities/`.

- *The Value of Precision Medicine*: `https://learn.genetics.utah.edu/content/precision/value/`.

- INCA model, the Netherlands, by Sanne Snoeijs, Verena Struckmann, Ewout van Ginneken: `http://www.icare4eu.org/pdf/INCA_Case_report.pdf`.

- The icons and personas used in the health experience and community figures in this book are courtesy of the Health and Youth Care Inspectorate of the Dutch Ministry of Health, Welfare and Sport, who kindly gave us their permission. The Inspectorate is supervising care networks and their position on care networks can be found in this position paper: *Good care in care networks* (`https://english.igj.nl/binaries/igj-en/documenten/publication/2018/08/16/good-care-in-care-networks/Good+care+in+care+networks+IGJ+May+2018+DEF+%28002%29.pdf`).

2
Exploring Relevant Technologies for Healthcare

An important way to learn is by playing with toys. MoM TiSH is going to let us play with some technology.

The theme for this chapter is technology possibilities for the platform. The impact of new and emerging technology on healthcare is huge. Digitalization is entering the world of clinicians, physicians, practitioners, caregivers, and increasingly, patients. Other major innovations include big data, **Artificial Intelligence (AI)**, robotics, and the **Internet of Things (IoT)**. In this chapter, we will explore the combined possibilities of new technologies, but always from the health experience perspective.

In this chapter, "relevant" means relevant to the transformation and shaping of the transformation team or community into a transformation task force. We will enrich the TiSH staircase with models for both the digitalization of healthcare and digitization into digital twins. We will introduce the **International Classification of Functioning, Disability, and Health (ICF)** as a reference model to understand medical digitization and discuss examples of networked care such as the **E-health Care Model (ECM)**, which makes it possible to deliver even complex care to the patient community, with the support of a platform.

Next, we will see how a company such as Amazon has embraced the health experience and utilized technology to provide better care. We will discuss what healthcare, in general, could learn from Amazon Care to provide a full healthcare experience during the patient's healthcare journey.

In this chapter, we're going to cover the following main topics:

- Exploring the impact of digitization
- Enabling virtual collaboration with telehealth
- Exploring the possibilities of AI, IoT, and robotics combined
- Learning from Amazon Care

Exploring the impact of digitization

To understand the impact of digitization, first, we have to study a worldwide model in medicine: the ICF.

> **Note**
>
> The ICF online browser can be found at `https://icd.who.int/dev11/l-icf/en`. This ICF browser is maintained by the **World Health Organization** (**WHO**) and endorsed by all member states. More information can be found at `https://www.who.int/standards/classifications/who-fic-maintenance`.

There's no need for medical training to comprehend it. In the following diagram, the ICF model describes how health conditions influence people and to what extent they can participate in society, given a specific condition:

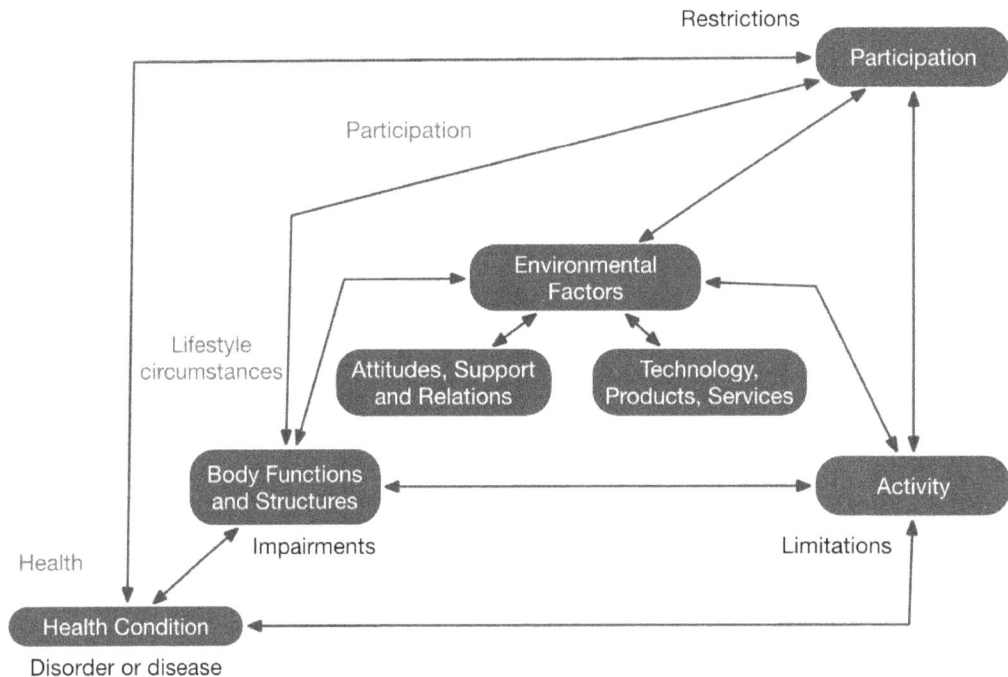

Figure 2.1 – The rearranged ICF model

Health is not just about the physical or mental condition; ICF also looks at health from a social perspective – for example, how well they fit into their community. The model shows how the overall health condition is defined by body functions and structures, activity, and the participation of a patient in relation to their circumstances of social and work lives and other environmental factors, such as the workplace, but also health insurance services.

True to our health experience, and referring to the TiSH treads, we have rearranged the ICF model with the personal circumstances of the patient's lifestyle at the center, participation in the upper-right corner as the outlook, and health in the lower-left corner as the prerequisite outcome of treatments for it. This way, it aligns with the upper three treads. With or without prior medical knowledge, it's easy to understand that a disorder or disease leads to impairment, limiting a patient's activities and resulting in restrictions on participation.

The online ICF browser provides a breakdown of the specific and detailed attributes that can all be recorded digitally. The digitization of these attributes is a prerequisite for an increased digitalization of care. For example, body function can be measured with the monitoring of vital signs or body structures via MRI or CT scans. **Environmental Factors**, **Activity**, and **Participation** are usually captured in conversations and reported in the **Electronic Patient Record** (**EPR**). Later in this chapter, we will learn that also these attributes can be digitized using technology. Try this for yourself and plot activity trackers in ICF.

With ICF, technology itself can also be related to improving the patient's life. Indeed, there's no denying that new technology has a tremendous impact on the provisioning and experience of healthcare. In ICF, environmental factors and the attitude towards the use of technology are explicated as attributes.

With this perspective, we can take a closer look at what the significant technology trends in healthcare are. These trends seem to concentrate around data, both on the edge where digitization takes place and in the cloud for secure storage and analytics. So far, the accompanying digital transformation or digitalization has led to the ability to collect, store, and access data in very efficient ways, for instance, using the cloud. The benefit of that is that care providers can rapidly share and retrieve data from each other. In theory, that should result in better patient care. We say, "in theory," because sharing data is not just about technology. There's a lot more that needs to be considered: regulations, compliance, privacy, and even the "willingness" or attitude to share data as a professional.

Understanding the impact of data exchange

However, the sharing of and interacting with data across platforms for healthcare provisioning is key in digital transformation as another aspect of data shows – big data. As it becomes easier to share and store data, it allows you to collect large amounts in clouds such as AWS, Microsoft Azure, and Google Cloud. This will especially benefit research, including epidemiological studies and clinical trials. Analyzing big datasets from various sources around the world will help in getting more accurate results in diagnostics and improve the methodologies of prevention and intervention.

Data is the source of every development. The clouds that we mentioned – AWS, Azure, and Google Cloud – are investing heavily in securely storing, accessing, and retrieving data. All of these platforms have developed special data lakes for healthcare propositions. They are using their cloud-specific data technology but adding functionality on top of it to get it compliant for use in healthcare. Some examples include AWS Healthlake and Azure for Healthcare.

> **TIP**
>
> There are many more cloud providers, but we will focus on the three major ones: AWS, Azure, and Google Cloud. Their healthcare solutions can be found at `https://aws.amazon.com/healthlake/` (AWS), `https://www.microsoft.com/en-us/industry/health/microsoft-cloud-for-healthcare` (Azure), and `https://cloud.google.com/healthcare` (Google Cloud).

These services are built on top of the technology of AWS, Azure, and Google Cloud, but with added functionality that targets services such as continuous patient monitoring, clinical analytics, and genomics research. This functionality supports the processes and protocol guidelines within the guardrails of regulations on security, privacy, safety, and costs.

This means that these services must be compliant with specific regulations, such as the **Health Insurance Portability and Accountability Act (HIPAA)** in the US and the **General Data Protection Regulation (GDPR)** or **European Health Data Space (EHDS)** in the EU.

As we will discuss in later chapters, interoperability between the stakeholders becomes key. This also means that they comply with standards in healthcare that enable data transfer and data exchange between different systems, such as standard APIs. For example, in healthcare, standard APIs include **Health Level (HL7)**, **Fast Healthcare Interoperability Resources (FHIR)**, and **Digital Imaging and Communications in Medicine (DICOM)** using the WHO Family of International Classifications, such as ICF. All of these standards describe how data, including medical images, can be exchanged between systems.

Now we can take a closer look at some of the major technological trends. Three trends seem to be game-changers in healthcare: AI, IoT, and robotics. We will discuss these in a separate section. Before we do that, we will look at networked care provisioning, which is made possible by the data exchange. In the final section, we will learn from Amazon Care how all of these technological trends and the health experience obsession fit together.

In the next section, we will discuss the impact of e-health (another word describing digital healthcare) as a form of technology to virtually connect the patient to care institutions and enhance virtual collaboration between care providers. Among others, we will look at an interesting and successful model that has been applied by the Danish Naerklinikken – the ECM – that redefines healthcare provisioning.

Enabling virtual collaboration with telehealth

One development has skyrocketed over the past few years, also caused by the global pandemic with the outbreak of COVID-19: virtual collaboration. The pandemic was a flywheel for the integrated collaboration between care providers enabled by digital technology.

Without any doubt, better collaboration between various care providers improves the level of care for the patient. This is not only about connecting the patient with the care provider, but also about the interconnection between care providers themselves, even in highly critical environments such as **Intensive Care Units (ICUs)**. Intensivists located in a central facility can monitor and coordinate the care of remote ICU beds, independent of where the beds are. The technology that they use for this is called tele-ICU. Of course, real-time data exchange is essential to be able to respond as quickly as possible when the patient shows signs of deterioration, and on-site intervention is required.

The virtual collaboration between medical professionals ensures that specialist expertise is more widely available. Exams and medical statuses can be shared among specialists for more holistic views on the diagnosis. This even includes the sharing of CT and MRI images for peer-to-peer reviews, advice, and education. Next, this data can be used to define the best treatment for a patient to obtain the best care.

The adoption and use of telehealth or e-health technology and virtual collaboration are expected to grow spectacularly in the coming years. The benefits are clear. First, it will make care more accessible. But through sharing knowledge, the quality of care will also improve. Additionally, telehealth applications will certainly increase provisioning capacity and drive down the costs of care.

Until this point, we talked about telehealth and even tele-ICUs. It would be better if we could prevent patients from ending up in hospitals. Modern technology also enables doctors to monitor patients remotely when they are still in the comfort of their own homes or if people are doing self-monitoring to stay healthy. Clinics around the world are piloting e-health applications and studying how this improves the comfort of their patients.

The outlook of participation with HeX

Having the ultimate health experience with the outlook of participating optimally in society is what **Health eXperience (HeX)** is about. It would be great if healthcare is individually directed by the people themselves from their desire to participate, whilst anticipating the possible restrictions caused by impairments that limit their activities. We could already think – or maybe dream – of the digitization of body and environment in a comprehensive digital twin and personalized avatar to foresee possible disorders and anticipate early lifestyle changes. We call this **Directed Care**.

However, before we get to this radical transformation of technology, we will revisit the **Integrated Care (INCA)** model and introduce the ECM of the Danisch Nearklinikken.

The essence of INCA is changing lifestyles and also addressing the community that the patient lives in. It's a new way of omniversal stepped care, providing the chronic care that we introduced briefly in the previous chapter as an example of a clinical provisioning model.

This approach is characterized by the following:

- Care is no longer provided in separate care programs as per the condition, but all health problems are together in one **Integrated Care Program** (**ICP**), in the context of the community along with all other important circumstances.

- The process flow is aiming at joint decision-making between the care providers and the patient for an optimum health experience, based on integrated findings from, for instance, consultations, physical examinations, and lab results done by different care providers.

- This leads to combined advice and jointly made decisions in an ICP, in a system that aggregates the data.

- After the creation of the ICP's the next steps and orders will be commenced: medication prescriptions, referrals, and additional diagnostic research. This will lead to a higher level of quality in the provisioning of care.

- There must be a patient tracking system in which both the care team and the patient are involved. Stakeholders need a single point of view in which all relevant information can be viewed.

- A patient portal is crucial to communicate with the patient.

MD Javier Asin has successfully implemented INCA in Surinam (Latin America), where it also helps optimize available and, often, scarce medical resources. Care is provided as close to the patient as possible within their community, and integrated care does not focus on only one condition but addresses the full health experience of the patient. Recently, it is more recognized that as body functions and structures always interact with each other, it could be beneficial for all treatments to include the whole health condition. INCA addresses this.

The key is that all data on the health condition and circumstances must be available for shared decision-making, requiring a high degree of integration – the integration of syntax, semantics, and pragmatic use in decision-making. Before realizing this level of digitization and digitalization, we have to learn how to do it in a less integrated way.

In the next section, we will take a closer look at a situation where care had to deal with legacy. Studied in Denmark, this was the ECM by the Naerklinikken.

Introducing the ECM

E-health is about bringing ever more complex care closer to the patient. Hospitals and other care facilities are in close reach of the patient using digital technologies. Clinics around the world have adopted models that show the benefits. An example is the Naerklinikken in Denmark, which works with ECM, embracing digital technologies to really focus on the patient's journey. The ECM model, as it is used by Naerklinikken, is shown in the following diagram:

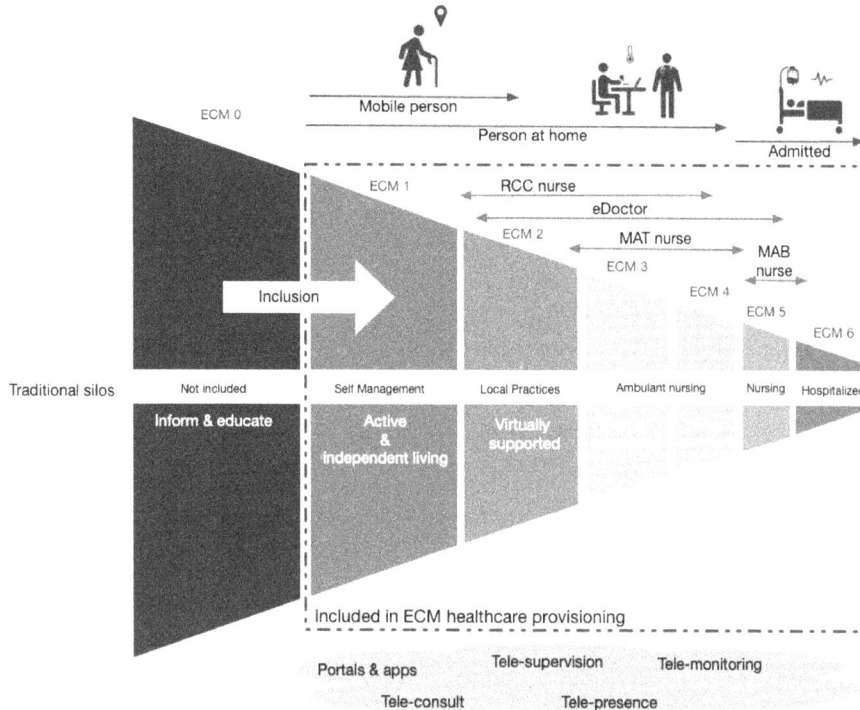

Derived from ECM Nærklinikken (Source: Søren Vingtoft)

Figure 2.2 – The ECM of Naerkliniiken in Denmark

The ECM organizes the required care activities in a different way. Instead of referring to the next care provider in the chain, the patient is included in a virtual clinic with all types of activities at their home, local practice, nursing home, and hospital included to form stepped healthcare provisioning. This is made possible because all different types of activities have access to the same information. Traditionally, local practices, ambulant nursing, nursing homes, and hospitals are different providers with their data mostly confined within the organization. With ECM having only one **Chief Medical Officer (CMO)**, these silos can be demolished.

But the main success factor was the interoperability and integration of data. The CMO, clinicians, and nurses had easy access to all of the patient data to make the best decisions based on it. Interoperability is the key technology and behavior to include from the start.

The second kind of technology to be included is telehealth functionalities: telemonitoring, tele-supervision, tele-consult, and telepresence. It literally makes healthcare provisioning boundaryless.

This results in the following **Stepped Care** approach:

- **ECM 0**: Persons who are healthy are informed to stay healthy and avoid risk factors to prevent illness or detect symptoms as early as possible.

- **ECM 1**: Once included, patients are to stay as mobile as possible to participate in society and receive, for example, medications that are specific to their condition and relevant self-monitoring equipment or apps, which also communicate directly with the **Response and Coordination Center** (**RCC**) of Naerklinikken for supervision.

- **ECM 2–4**: The patient is less or no longer mobile but receives care at home. As soon as an acute deterioration is experienced by the patient, or it is signaled by the telemonitoring equipment, the RCC responds 24/7. Either in a purely virtual way (ECM 2) with tele-supervision or, if necessary, by sending a local specially trained **Mobile Acute Nurse** (**MAN**), to investigate further (ECM 3). If necessary, the treatment starts in the patient's own home (ECM 4). The *eDoctor* of the Naerklinikken supervises in the background via tele-consult and, if required, with telepresence via smart glasses worn by the nurse.

- **ECM 5**: If necessary, the patient is admitted to a local bed unit in the municipality, where the patient receives 24/7 treatment and care from the nursing staff.

- **ECM 6**: If the situation still deteriorates, the patient is admitted to the hospital.

ECM is a model for redesigned sustainable healthcare on a small scale, using the various modern technologies that we discussed in the previous sections. The model shows how you shape healthcare around a patient, using relevant technology to do so, and at the same time, substantially lower the costs of care.

The first results of the studies at Naerklinikken show that 70 to 80 percent of all acute aggravations of patients can be handled successfully through virtual communication such as portals and telehealth in ECM 1 and ECM 2. Another 10 to 15 percent can be treated in ECM 3 and ECM 4, where the patient is still at home and visiting nurses are supported by telemonitoring. A very small remaining group must still be admitted to the hospital in ECM 6.

There are two major benefits to using this model. First, the patient can be treated at home for a longer time, which is more convenient and comfortable for the patient. Secondly, studies have shown a decrease in care costs of approximately 8,000 USD per year per patient.

Therefore, on a small scale, Naerklinikken forms a redesigned healthcare model, which is characterized by an integrated organization aimed at coordination, supported using e-health. Care providers in Norway, Canada, and the Netherlands are currently adopting this model.

However, as we will discuss in later chapters, transforming from a siloed legacy is not easy.

Connecting the hospital to home with virtual care at scale

In the previous section, we saw that technologies are emerging to interact with patients in their own homes, monitoring their health conditions. This greatly impacts the way healthcare can be organized. Telehealth and e-health technology will enable greater possibilities for patients to connect with their care provisioning and vice versa. It will make care better and more accessible and, at the same time, grant providers opportunities to guide patients in their lifestyle, preventing health issues.

The COVID-19 pandemic accelerated these developments. To avoid the risk of transmission of the SARS-CoV-2 virus, doctors and other medical staff turned to technology to see their patients through *virtual visits* and by monitoring them remotely. Reducing the risk of transmission was key and also avoiding hospitals from being flooded with COVID patients. Hospital resources became scarcer than ever before.

Remote patient monitoring and e-consultations are here to stay even after the pandemic. They have proven to be more convenient for a patient: in many cases, the patient can stay safely at home, while being monitored remotely.

The pandemic has proven that digital health solutions can be implemented at scale. This opens great possibilities to make healthcare more available and accessible for millions of people around the world who, today, lack that access. The WHO calculates that half of the world's population does not have access to quality healthcare. Without transformation to more sustainable models, this number is likely to rise to 5 billion people by 2030. Therefore, the WHO urges healthcare organizations and providers to implement digital solutions that enable that access for everyone.

In short, we need technology that connects the homes of millions to hospitals and clinics around the world. With e-consultations, remote monitoring, and virtual collaboration between medical professionals, it's possible to provide healthcare at scale, anywhere, anytime.

However, developing this type of patient-centric healthcare provisioning requires a different mindset and substantial resources from the IT sector.

Urgency, such as a pandemic, is certainly helping as no other way is available. To envisage how the first steps can be made, we will study how it fits in situations of more traditional healthcare provisioning.

Working with the four treads of networked care in TiSH

We have learned about the goal of participating in omniversal HeX, integrated care as a way to make lifestyle part of the treatment, and ECM as a stepped care model to collaborate in the treatment of health conditions. The treatment itself consists of several typical actions such as intake, diagnostics, and treatment. Usually, these actions are managed by the patient or a professional, respectively called self-management or case management. This is shown in the following diagram:

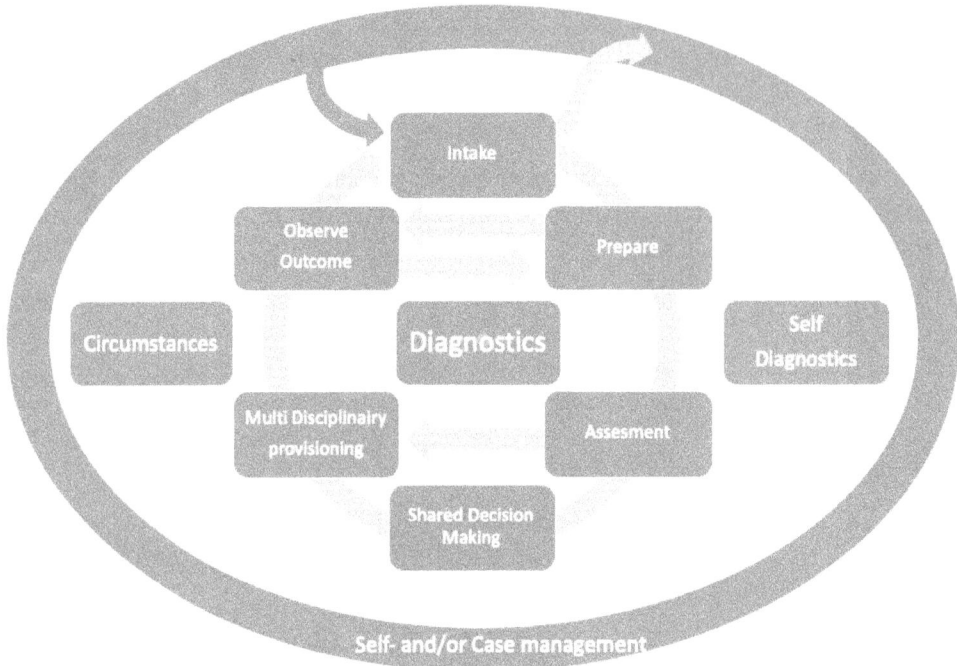

Figure 2.3 – Self-management and case management

The preceding diagram shows how the generic activities of healthcare are summarized to realize a patient's journey. Present-day communication is used to inform each other on the planning of consultations and treatments, medical data collection, and referring to other organizations and disciplines, which are done in accordance with the standing procedures.

When you or a representative is experiencing a disorder, an intake is planned, and further actions are prepared in accordance with treatment protocols for assessment of the disorder in terms of body functions and structures. Based on the diagnostics of either the assessment or further tests, decisions are made about treatments. Treatments are provided and observed until the outcome is satisfactory, after which a discharge from the hospital or ambulatory treatment is executed.

Each activity has its own digital system to support the activity. The digitization and digitalization of each of these activities are the first steps toward the true digital provisioning of healthcare interaction. It's the starting point for networked care.

Four types of networked care

We discussed the general impact of digitalization on healthcare with emerging technological possibilities for data exchange, virtual collaboration, and e-health, resulting in four distinctive ways of networked care enabled by technology. The following diagram shows them with the assigned symbols or icons that we will use later in this book:

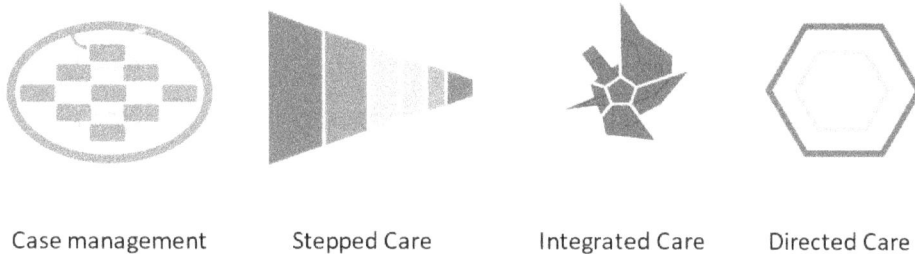

| Case management | Stepped Care | Integrated Care | Directed Care |

Figure 2.4 – Four treads of networked care

We will explain the preceding diagram from left to right. It starts with the case management we just described in which care activities are digitized, enabling communication between the activities. Next is **Stepped Care**, where collaboration between several disciplines in different locations or teams can provide continuous treatment following the actual condition of the patient and making sure that the patient can stay as active as possible.

Once **Stepped Care** is performed well for one condition or disease, others can follow until a point is reached where it becomes necessary to cooperate between the disciplines and involve the circumstances of the community. If **Integrated Care** has been mastered, it is possible to organize **Directed Care** to direct the care and provide solutions that enable participation in society, as desired by individuals. This sequence gives us a clear development path for the transformation to networked care.

We have studied the impact technologies can and will have on the digitalization of healthcare networks. In the next sections, we will study three underlying game-changers in healthcare in the context of this evolving networked care: AI, **robotics**, and **IoT**.

Exploring the possibilities of AI, IoT, and robotics

The platform of communities and systems that we foresee are using a combination of different technologies. In fact, no single technology will be a game-changer on its own. They have to be integrated, as demonstrated in the following figure:

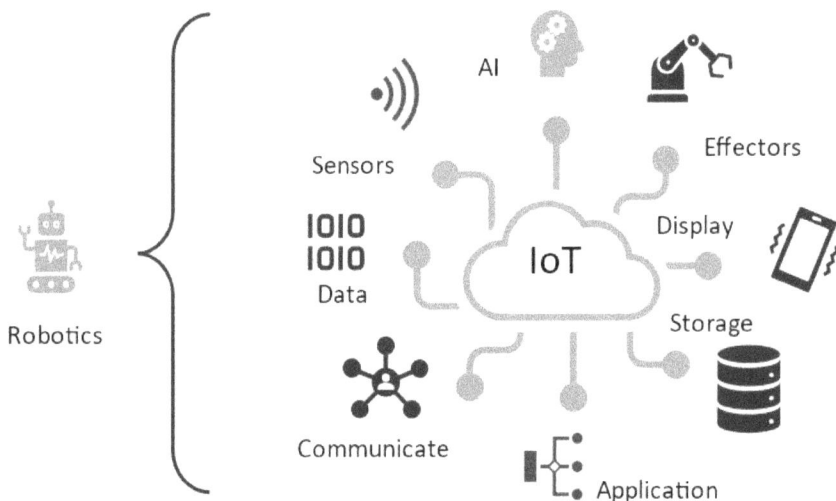

Figure 2.5 – Integrating technologies

However, IoT, AI, and robotics do bring more traditional technologies together to perform far more than each technology could on its own. **Interoperability and Integration (I&I)** are keys that we will address in *Chapter 3*, *Unfolding the Complexity of Transformation*.

We will keep that in mind in the following exploration of the three selected technologies, along with the fact that there are far more technologies that are used in healthcare.

The possibilities of AI

AI is perceived to be a game-changer in healthcare. In the previous section, we briefly talked about the major cloud providers that have developed specific solutions for healthcare. Without exception, all of these solutions rely on AI. Before we learn why AI has a great impact on healthcare, we need to understand what AI is and what it's not.

AI uses vast amounts of data, computational calculations of algorithms, continuous analytics, and deep learning to provide professionals with accurate data as input for clinical decision-making. We deliberately use the word "input" here since AI is never a replacement for the work and responsibility of a professional. The professional – a radiologist, clinician, researcher, practitioner, or surgeon – will always have the final say in any decision.

The next step is to elaborate on the use cases for healthcare and its provisioning. We can think of the following:

- **Diagnostics**: Algorithms can help to detect diseases. AI is already widely accepted in the diagnosis of cancer and adding value to the interpretation of critical findings in medical imaging. One example is prostate cancer, where AI can help diagnose cancer spots already in a very early stage (for instance, by using heat maps) and set the accurate so-called Gleason score to determine how aggressive the cancer is. Additionally, AI is used to flag abnormalities; help to predict the outcomes and the prognosis of chronic diseases. Another example is smartwatches or home sensors with vital signs and motion monitoring, where algorithms can detect trends such as deteriorating mobility or acute anomalies such as falling or irregular heart rates.

- **Treatments**: AI is used to predict the outcomes of the treatment, but also to define the right treatment plan. This is the field of personalized treatment, not where one patient is just like another. Persons are unique and might respond differently to treatments. Personalized treatment and personalized medicine are expected to improve the patient's life drastically. AI and machine learning can help to discover the specific characteristics that indicate certain responses to treatment. Again, this is heavily reliant on data. AI will compare the outcomes of the treatments with patient references to get more accurate results. For example, algorithms are now used for the precision tuning of insulin pumps.

- **Clinical path optimization**: The clinical pathway sets out the journey for patients with a specific disease, defining the clinical steps that must be taken to come to the desired result in the treatment of the disease. Pathways require scheduling, but this is a complex process in healthcare. First, clinicians must have a good understanding of the patient's overall condition. That defines the following steps in the process for which appointments need to be scheduled, varying from a scan (diagnosis) to treatment, what information to use in shared decision-making with the patients, and monitoring the patient after an intervention.

  At every stage, the appropriate resources must be available in time: think of the availability of the scanner and the operating radiologist, the surgery and surgeon, the ICU and skilled ICU staff, the transport from hospital to home, and the nurses to look after the patient after being hospitalized. During this process, medical indicators must be closely monitored since they can affect the pathway and the clinical choices. AI can help in optimizing the planning of resources and ensure that patients get the right attention at the right time. Planning resources are often routine tasks that can consume a lot of the professional's time and, in fact, distract them from the patient's needs. For instance, studies have shown that 25 percent of the work in radiology departments could be automated. This work mostly concerns the scheduling of routine exams.

- **Health analytics on populations**: We can learn a lot by analyzing groups of patients over time and by viewing behaviors and conditions in specified populations. Defining these populations is referred to as clustering. Such a cluster can be a group of patients with a specific chronic condition. By tracking this group, we can learn about the effects of health plans and provided care. The goal is to improve health outcomes by analyzing vast amounts of data in a specific group of patients and, at the same time, reduce care costs since the analysis will show how care can be "adjusted" for more efficiency and better results.

  An example of this methodology is the **Adjusted Clinical Group (ACG) system** by Johns Hopkins. AI and machine learning are major accelerators for getting results from the data, through predictive modeling, performance management, identifying trends and opportunities to improve diagnostics and treatment, and tracking and forecasting diseases.

> Tip
> We recommend learning more about the ACG system of Johns Hopkins at `hopkinsacg.org`.

Let's recap why we need to transform into more sustainable healthcare. We discussed the challenges in the previous chapter: we will be faced with growing numbers of patients and patients who will need care for a longer time. At the same time, we have a growing shortage of medical staff. This includes doctors and care staff. AI can certainly lift some of the burdens, as we have seen in the preceding examples; for example, with faster and more accurate diagnoses and efficient treatments.

The possibilities of robotics

AI without an effector like a robot to act is useful for decision support. However, with an effector, we arrive in the world of robotics. Robots are everywhere, and they are certainly emerging in healthcare. They vary from the Da Vinci robot used for surgery to packing robots for medication, medication dispensers, nursing robots, and even social robots. In this section, we will study some of these robots and, in particular, how they improve the life of the patient:

- **Surgical robots**: Da Vinci is an example of such a robot. Da Vinci Surgery has delivered surgical systems around the world, including the Da Vinci Xi, which enables **Robotic Assisted Surgery for Patients**. Here, the keyword is **assisted** since the robot is not able to perform surgery on its own: it's assisting the surgeon in performing the procedure, although the development of autonomous systems is evolving.

  The biggest benefit of robots is the precision of their operations: they can perform complex surgeries without making large incisions, especially when they are driven by AI-enabled navigation. The benefit for the patient is that operations are less impactful, and recovery is likely to proceed faster, with less burden on the healthcare system as a whole.

- **Service robots**: Packing robots and dispensers are examples of service robots. In essence, these robots take care of routine and primarily logistical tasks. These robots do operate autonomously in most cases, relieving care staff from these routine tasks. The benefit for patients is that care staff will have more time to focus on care and the patient. The near future promises Asimo-type general-purpose robots to assist in daily medical tasks. Boston Dynamics, Samsung, and Tesla are already on it.

- **Social robots**: This might still be unchartered territory, but social robots will definitively play a role in future healthcare, especially in long-term and mental care. For instance, we can see good practices in the treatment of Alzheimer's patients. Social robots interact with patients and help improve the well-being of the patient by exercising movements or cognitive functions such as concentration, orientation, speech, and memory.

Robots are mostly task-based and work alongside and with humans. As such, the application of robots can be used in any tread of the transformation. One side effect is that robots have many sensors that result in more digitization and a better model for the digital twin. Sensors are, very often, embedded in IoT, which we will discuss in the following section.

The possibilities of IoT in healthcare

E-health, in its contemporary form, is the application of IoT in the healthcare business. The same reference architecture and technologies as the following one from Azure can be used to scale ECM or INCA-type healthcare provisioning:

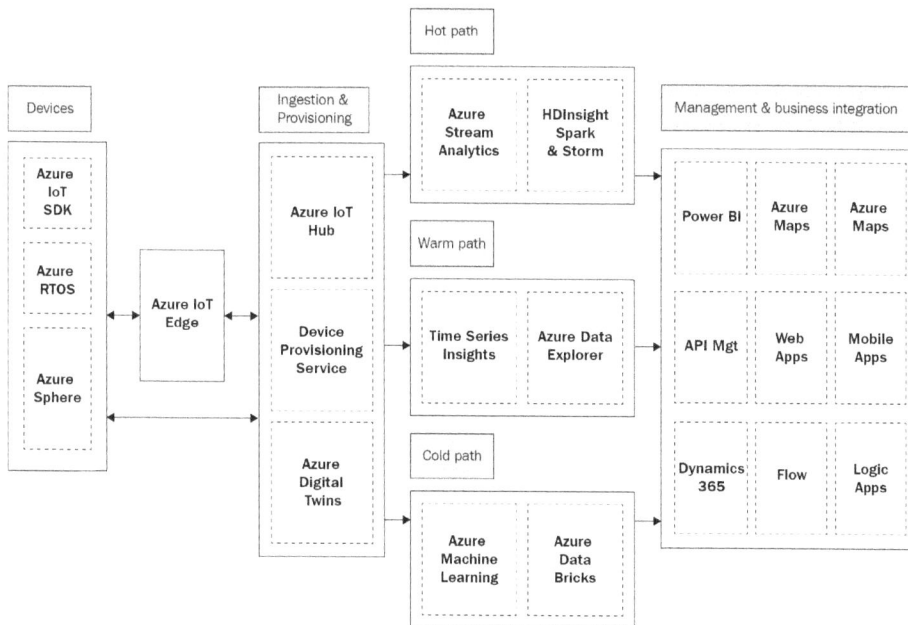

Figure 2.6 – The IoT reference architecture (Azure)

Healthcare IoT devices are typical sensors, such as vital sign sensors, alarm buttons, motion detectors, and effectors such as medication dispensers, smart locks, smart glasses worn by visiting nurses, and also many smart devices such as smartwatches, smartphones, and home automation systems that can be used in a concerted way for healthcare provisioning.

Developments are rapid, and we advise finding websites or communities to follow the trends in this area on a weekly or even daily basis. Functions such as telemonitoring, tele-supervision, telepresence, and tele-consultations can be realized with IoT technology. You can imagine that many IoT devices can measure a lot of the conditions and circumstances to build a dense digital picture, for instance, the digital twin.

But there are also downsides to internet-connected devices.

Security is an issue here, and currently, getting attention from governments to regulate the security of home automation and IoT is a challenge. We will discuss this and other regulations later in this book.

We talked about the possibilities of emerging technology. We also discussed how this technology might improve the life of the patient. So, how far are we from really adopting this mature and emerging tech? And are there companies that have already embraced this completely in their transformation and include this technology in a new model of healthcare? We studied the case of Naerklinikken in Denmark, which has proven that, with e-health, it's possible to provide high-quality care outside of hospitals.

Applying technology in networked care and TiSH

We introduced the models for understanding how technology can drive transformation, as mentioned in the first chapter of this book. Now we are going to put them into the perspective of the TiSH staircase. The highest step aims for participation, where the objectives can be expressed in terms of the ICF model. Lifestyle objectives can be expressed in terms of environmental factors, body functions, and activities, and health objectives in terms of the health condition of the ICF model. We use the upper three tiers of the TiSH staircase for setting and deriving the objectives. We classify the treatment tier with the type of networked care, case management, stepped care, integrated care, and directed care. From there, we can use TiSH as follows: case management for treatments, stepped care for health objectives, integrated care for lifestyle objectives, and directed care for participation objectives.

We put it in this order, as each next tread becomes more complex with more parties involved and more factors to consider. Each tread requires a better understanding of digitization and digitalization. It starts with having information available digitally, being able to exchange data, activating effectors such as a medication dispenser, using sensors on patients, collecting environmental data with IoT, analyzing the data with AI, and using all of this in autonomous robots. The message is that the higher the objectives are on a larger scale, the more advanced technology has to be to fulfill the objectives.

A visual overview is provided in the following diagram:

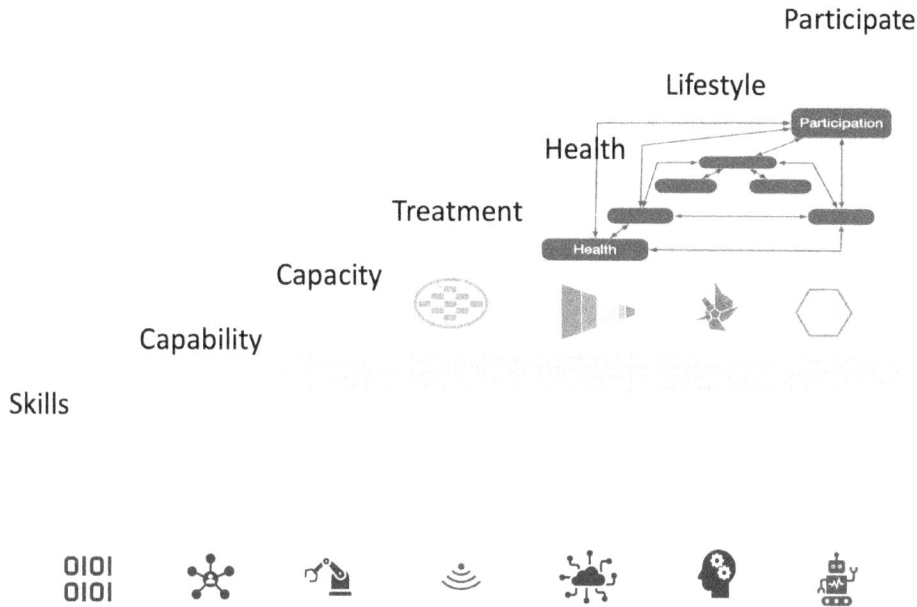

Figure 2.7 – TiSH, ICF, networked care, and technologies

It starts with learning to digitize care activities, communicating digitally in teams, having enough capacity to use robotics as medicine dispensers or social robots, observing the patient in real time with sensors to guide treatments, using IoT to collect environmental data and connecting across care providers for stepped care, using AI to its full extent to support a lifestyle with integrated care, and finally, applying autonomous robots to fully utilize all the gathered data for the best health experience and outlook on participation. Every step creates more complexity in the integration and interoperability of the different technologies and the provisioning of care.

In the next section, we will look at one other example. In this case, it's not a healthcare organization, but a company that adopted a new model of providing healthcare for its employees and is fully worker-centric in the worker's community of the company. The question we should ask is what could we learn from this company, Amazon Care?

Learning from Amazon Care

We live in a world that seems to be ever more reliant on technology. In fact, this chapter has been all about technology. In the previous sections, we explored various new technologies, the possibilities they bring, and their relevance in healthcare. But so far, we haven't connected the dots to the health experience. All this technology doesn't have any value if we don't connect it in the right way: with the patient at center stage.

Patient-centric means that the patient is at the center of it all, surrounded by care, and able to access cures. We learned that this is the essence of the HeXagon, which we introduced in the first chapter, to model the health experience. HeX is provided through enabling and supporting relevant technologies such as telehealth in remote patient monitoring. In turn, telehealth, such as patient monitoring, is enabled through data technology and connectivity. Let's explore HeX a bit further:

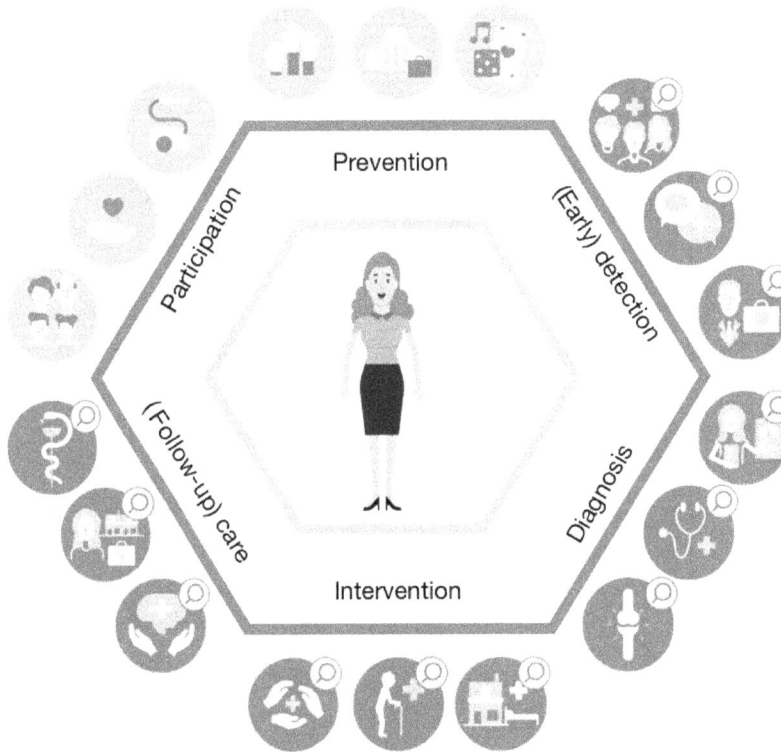

Figure 2.8 – HeX: The Health eXperience hexagon

The patient is at the core of the HeXagon. The various activities of care are depicted in the first ring: prevention, (early) detection, diagnosis, intervention, (follow-up) care, and participation. All of these activities are supported by specific healthcare services, either in clinical settings or at home. Of course, participation is the most important activity in this model: the other activities should enable participation. This is the golden rule of the HeXagon: *the value of a good health condition is to be able to engage in activities to participate in society.*

As we have seen with ECM and the previous section on technologies, the I&I of data is the key. This is symbolized by the outer blue line and inner yellow line. The outer blue line symbolizes the medical and health data, and the inner yellow line represents the coordination between all actors in the community involved in health provisioning.

> **Note**
>
> The **Blue Line** concept was first introduced in the Village of the Future Workshop at the MIE2012 in Pisa, Italy. Afterward, it was developed at the PCSI, in 2015, in The Hague, where the Blue Line Statement 2015 was presented to the alderman of healthcare. It starts with the following: *In order to achieve meaningful improvements in the health of the population, it is essential to understand the combination of health and social care issues for people.*

If we take a closer look at participation, then we could learn from Amazon Care, a company that has put theory into practice.

The model starts with the philosophy that the employee is able to work. Reduced work performance and sick leave are undesirable for both the employee and the employer. Therefore, Amazon takes care that both the contextual factors, such as the workplace and the employee's health condition are optimal. Put simply, the goal is to have the employee participate as much as possible.

The value is in participation. In this case, the direct business case for the efforts is formed by the relationship between the employee and the employer. Medical attention is aimed at the desired level of participation: it balances the desire to stay and become active again for the employer with the time required to recover from an undesired health condition.

Now, where does emerging technology play a role in this? In Amazon, it plays a huge role. In fact, it is comparable to the ECM and INCA models that we discussed in the previous sections. By using technology, care is "tuned" to the needs of the patient. Or, in the words of Amazon, *get the care you need in seconds, in all the moments that matter*. That's the second insight: companies such as Amazon are extremely good at customizing services to the needs, wishes, and expectations of their customers. That's what healthcare, in general, could learn from Amazon Care.

The final insight: technology is the enabler. It provides the possibilities for change. Amazon Care starts with an app, making it possible to schedule virtual visits with clinicians 7 days a week, 365 days a year. Patients can chat with clinicians. The data stays with the patient and is transferable to any provider. If needed, Amazon Care arranges follow-up care at home and, if required, with dedicated care teams. Remember ECM?

Let's summarize the lessons that we could learn from Amazon Care:

- Apply the principles of customer satisfaction rigorously (patient-obsessed)
- Apply the anyplace, anytime, anywhere logistics to healthcare provisioning
- Make sure you have a direct business case, and not just an indirect social business case where value streams are disconnected and must be heavily regulated

Chapter 1, *Understanding (the Need for) Transformation*, was about the urgency to transform healthcare. This chapter discussed the possibilities of technology in this transformation. By now, you should have a good understanding of the possibilities and level of complexity that are faced in transforming healthcare and shaping our transformation task force. In the next chapter, we will try to unfold this complexity in more detail.

Summary

In this chapter, the central theme was possibilities. This included possibilities related to health and the ability to be active and participate, which we learned to define in terms of the ICF model. We learned that technology can enable networked care evolving from case management in a network, stepped care, integrated care, and directed care. We explored the possibilities of relevant technology in healthcare and discussed the use of big data, telehealth, AI, robotics, and IoT. These technologies are perceived to be game-changers in healthcare.

Telehealth has skyrocketed during the pandemic: more clinics are using e-health technology to connect to their patients but also to encourage virtual collaboration between professionals. We learned that access to data is key in almost every technology. We need data to analyze and get better results in diagnosis, treatment, clinical path optimization, and care.

In this chapter, we took a more detailed look at two relevant best practices: the ECM of the Danish Naerklinikken and Amazon Care. Both come from the same angle: the patient is at the core of both models. The models aim to get the best care to the patient at the most convenient times. We saw that what we learned can be applied to the transformation toward sustainable healthcare or TiSH.

In the next chapter, we will dive into the complexity of transforming healthcare systems by, first, studying the regulatory aspects, the role of the different stakeholders, and how they might be disrupted during the transformation. Additionally, we will look at the roles of the major technology providers and what they bring to the table.

Further reading

- Body of knowledge for ICF, International Classification of Functioning, Disability, and Health: `https://apps.who.int/classifications/icfbrowser/`
- Google blog on federated learning: `https://ai.googleblog.com/2017/04/federated-learning-collaborative.html`
- *Working backwards* by Colin Bryar and Bill Carr, St. Martins PR, 2021
- *Social care informatics as an essential part of holistic health care: A call for action* by Michael Rigby, International Journal of Medical Informatics

Unfolding the Complexity of Transformation

3

To get more understanding, playing with toys is not enough, we need to learn the complexities. MoM TiSH will lead us to some education on complexity.

The theme for this chapter is defining the *complexity* of healthcare. In the first two chapters, we saw that healthcare is subject to huge changes and that requires transformation. Transformation is complex and requires new disciplines to address it and realize the desired platform. We introduced the systems engineers and community builders needed for this in the transformation task force.

Systems engineers need to define the complexity of networked care using the decomposition and classification of less complex components. This chapter will provide you with models for describing the complexity characteristics of networked care on the development path toward higher treads in the transformation and describe how it affects all the systems in the healthcare sector.

We will learn about the policies and regulations that form guardrails in healthcare. We will also see how traditional healthcare provisioning based on guidelines is more focused on the output of a particular process and not the integrated health outcome for patients.

We will look at how community builders use different methodologies to define the real value for all stakeholders, such as the revenue for care providers and a better health experience for the patient. We will learn how to discover this value by listening to the voice of the patient and integrating processes in the design, development, and operations of healthcare solutions. This is the start of implementing DevOps4Care for the **Transformation into Sustainable Healthcare (TiSH)**.

In this chapter, we're going to cover the following topics:

- Defining complexity

- Exploring policies and regulations

- Understanding the value of care with DevOps principles

- Understanding technology in complex systems

- Understanding the role of major technology enablers

Defining complexity

In the first two chapters, we introduced TiSH and the upper four treads consisting of networked care. We learned about case management, stepped care, integrated care, and directed care. Each tread introduced more technology for digitization such as robotics, IoT, and AI to get closer to the optimum health experience. The complexity increases rapidly with each tread. But what is complexity?

Luckily, defining complexity is not so complex if we involve system engineers. Complexity in our context is the characteristics and resulting behavior of the healthcare system in which many components with multiple relations interact in multiple ways and follow certain guardrails and guidelines. It would suffice for us to concentrate on the characteristics of components and the relations and interactions between the components for now. What can we learn from systems engineers?

Complexity emerges from the many possible interactions. This follows the essence of the definition of complexity given by the **International Council of Systems Engineering** (**INCOSE**) body of knowledge – *A measure of how difficult it is to understand how a system will behave or to predict the consequences of changing it* (Sheard and Mostashari, 2009).

> Tip
>
> The **Systems Engineering Body of Knowledge** (**SEBoK**) maintained by the aforementioned INCOSE provides a guide to key knowledge sources and references in systems engineering. We will refer to this body of knowledge several times in this book for further information. You can search for the word complexity and follow the discussion on this topic. More information is available at `https://www.sebokwiki.org/wiki/Guide_to_the_Systems_Engineering_Body_of_Knowledge_(SEBoK)`.

Where does healthcare stand in complexity on a scale of one to ten? It depends, of course. Prescribing paracetamol and getting it from the pharmacy is straightforward. Let's say that's a 2. Having a hip replacement and going through an MRI scan, surgery, and rehabilitation with medication quickly becomes much more complex. We'll call this a 5. But if we zoom out and look at the supply chain of the MRI scanner or paracetamol, then we enter the global supply chain. So, that's easily a 7. If we include the financial aspects, such as reimbursement, we reach an 8, and if we do that over someone's life span, we are at a 9. So, where is the 10? Imagine doing all of this on the moon. With NASA's upcoming Artemis missions at the time of writing, maybe it's something we can look forward to.

Describing the characteristics of networked care in terms of its components, relations, and interactions will help us to create a common understanding of transformation.

As we are not the first to describe complex systems, we can look for descriptions and definitions that are already available. By combining several of them, we get a specific understanding of networked care in terms of these interactions, relations, and components. Here, we will present two applicable models to describe the complexity of networked care in terms of interaction and relation.

Defining interaction

Interactions are needed to get information for some form of decision-making to agree on how to take the next steps. We can use the **foresee (4C)** model for that. It provides guidance on the best way to make a decision. Although, we have to take decisions in order to reach the goals that we have set, reaching these goals, as we have seen, might be influenced by changes in health conditions or environmental factors. Hence, we need to be able to adjust these decisions based on the acquired knowledge and come up with new insights. There are many variations of the 4C model, but we define it as follows:

- **Communications**: The interaction of ideas, opinions, and feelings in order to reach a mutual understanding of a topic and decide individually

- **Coordination**: The joint effort of integrating activities to enable the efficient allocation of resources within or between organizations and its team and team members

- **Control**: The management of setting goals and standards, measuring performance against the standards to validate whether goals will be achieved, and if needed, taking corrective action

- **Command**: The process of directly giving orders

We can characterize the four types of networked care as per the 4C model. It's obvious that *communication* always takes place right from the start with the case manager taking decisions. With stepped care, *coordination* becomes more relevant to decide which step is required. Integrated care requires *control* on which condition to treat first. Directed care is about the patient and their condition directing a *command* about what care is required in the first place.

In healthcare, we will see that decision-making differs for each stakeholder. In a heavily regulated industry such as healthcare, governmental bodies set standards in terms of compliance requirements. Insurance companies issue direct orders in terms of reimbursable costs. Care teams will need coordination to get things done. In all these cases, communication is essential since every stakeholder requires information to gain knowledge before any decision can be taken.

Defining relations

With respect to the relations between the different types of networked care, we were inspired by ISO 21839, 2019 to name the four stages of networked organizations with the definitions of **Systems of Systems (SoS)**. SoS are used for systems containing many systems interacting with other systems. Think of the communication between two hospitals with each having its own system for electronic patient records. These combinations of interacting systems can be characterized as follows:

- **Ad hoc**: The healthcare network lacks a central management authority and a centrally agreed-upon purpose for the ad-hoc created SoS. This type of SoS relies on mostly unseen mechanisms – for instance, underlying legislation or de facto industry standards. They may emerge in large-scale systems.

- **Collaborative**: The component systems of each provider interact more or less voluntarily to fulfill agreed-upon network purposes. Here, mechanisms of enforcement and maintained agreements play a role since stakeholders collectively decide how to provide or revoke services.

- **Acknowledged**: The healthcare network has recognized objectives, a designated manager, and resources for the joined SoS. Underlying systems still have their respective owners and own objectives, funding, development, and sustainment approaches. Changes are triggered and sustained through cooperative agreements between the SoS and the systems.

- **Directed**: The SoS is created and managed by the healthcare network to fulfill its purpose and achieve objectives where underlying systems become an integrated part of the SoS, whilst components of systems can still operate independently. However, the SoS is the leading, overarching system.

This derived definition (the original generic formulation can be found in the SEBoK) will help us to define the stages of the transformation.

> **Tip**
>
> **ISO** – the **International Organization for Standardization** – and regional or national standards are a great repository of knowledge anyway and are easy to use for defining a common reference.

It is quite plausible that as part of the development path, a network starts ad hoc as a virtual network and progresses toward being a directed network. It's the case manager that forms ad-hoc networks depending on what an episode of care requires. In stepped care, the collaboration between the systems of each provider is required for coordination. Integrated care needs designated management of the systems to stay in control. For directed care, the patient must be able to trust that the systems are fit for the specific purpose to predict their future health condition and circumstances, as mentioned in the **International Classification of Functioning, Disability and Health** (**ICF**) model.

So, what interacting and related systems are we talking about? That is what we will define next.

Defining systems

Healthcare provisioning consists of many activities with supporting systems and their components. We define the characteristics of the systems and components based on the activities within healthcare that we mentioned in *Chapter 2*, *Exploring Relevant Technologies for Healthcare*, where we introduced the four types of networked care. Using the ICF model, these activities have a clear purpose (or main characteristic) related to health, lifestyle, and participation.

Let's start with the activities of case management:

- **Intake** after a decision made by the patient based on their perceived health condition
- **Prepare** the pending care episode using the relevant medical history
- **Assessments** in triage using (self-)diagnostics, including registered circumstances
- **Decision-making** as the next step to either end the episode, provide more diagnostics, or commence treatment
- **Providing treatment** or other intervention
- **Observation** of outcomes

Each of these activities uses specific systems to do things such as measure vital signs, record the findings, order diagnostics, plan staff, manage reimbursement, provide CT scans, or prepare for an operation, rehabilitation, or nursing. The specific systems include **electronic patient records** (**EPRs**) and **enterprise resource planning** (**ERP**), with modules for **human resource management** (**HRM**), **quality assurance** (**QA**), and **business intelligence** (**BI**) for financial control, among others. This results in a distinct application landscape for each organization. These landscapes can be very extensive and complex on their own. It's a SoS with architecture and governance.

For now, it suffices to know that the activities we defined as components have some internal structure.

Adding to the aforementioned activities, the case manager uses a system for communication with the different providers in the care network. This system can also comprise several applications – for example, several apps on the mobile phone of the patient. That is a system too, used mostly for communication.

With stepped care, the different landscapes of the different providers and the case manager are connected for the coordination of activities between the providers. This requires a coordinating system to connect the systems of the different care providers. This system is not necessarily a physical system – it can also be a coordination agreement to adhere to certain standards on the interoperability of systems.

With integrated care, the joint management of the interoperability and integration of systems is a system of its own. This is more than a coordination agreement; it requires a control activity to be managed. Think of joint DevOps activities and the systems they need.

Directed care requires yet another activity – the governance of all systems must ensure that people can rely on the availability of all the required systems for the optimum health experience as defined by society.

Let's recap what we have presented so far. To describe complexity, we learned how to characterize complexity based on the type of interaction between components, the relationship between components, and the components themselves for each type of networked care using the 4C model. See the visualization in the following table:

Networked Care Components	Interaction	Relation
Directed Care Governance	Command	Directed
Integrated Care Integration	Control	Acknowledged
Stepped Care Agreement	Coordination	Collaboration
Case management Communication Intake Prepare Assess Decide Provide Observe	Communication	Virtual

Table 3.1 – The structural complexity characteristics of networked care

Exploring policies and regulations

Policies and regulations are determined by governments and their institutes. Although it differs for each country or region, it is possible to recognize certain elements, whether a national health service, such as the **NHS** in the UK, municipal, as in Finland, or regulated to some extent via insurance companies, as in a lot of countries in the European Union, or via the employer, as practiced in the US.

Policies and regulations set the guardrails for the development of solutions. Hence, we need to start with this. There's no escaping or working around policies and regulations – we simply have to deal with them. In this section, we will explore policies, regulations, principles, and the various stakeholders that have to work with these **rules of engagement** in healthcare. We will learn how these rules are crucial in the delivery and transformation of healthcare.

We call these the rules of engagement, a military term that explains the internal rules for defense forces that set the guardrails for the circumstances, conditions, levels, and methods that justify the use of force by defense resources. These can be derived from internal agreements or rules set by law. As we are defending our health, it's a metaphor you can use to make sense of policies, regulations, and the behavior of stakeholders in healthcare.

Policies and regulations set the guardrails for the circumstances, conditions, levels, treatments, and other types of interventions that necessitate care being given to patients. It's not just the opinion, experience, skills, or judgment of a clinician or the feelings of a patient that set these conditions and circumstances. There are laws, policies, principles, standards, budgets, and even public opinions set by the media that define the conditions for the delivery and innovation of healthcare. Safety, privacy, cost, and above all, value are some of the most important themes here.

The following list contains some examples of these rules of engagement in healthcare, but is by no means exhaustive:

- Policies on what is in the scope of healthcare. Think of plastic surgery, the prevention of becoming ill, birth control, alternative medicine, certain treatments that only concern a small group, or the way palliative treatments should be done. These can be ethical issues and are influenced by politics.

- The scientific proof of treatments and medicine. This is used to define what is referred to as claims in medicine. The formal value of treatments and medicine.

- The cost of healthcare. Think of the huge cost of resources and the time spent developing medicine.

- Inspection and audits on quality and safety. An example is a recent bill in the US that calls for a **Software Bill of Materials** (**SBOM**) for 510(k)-eligible products. 510(k) is the technical dossier required by the US **Food and Drug Administration** (**FDA**) that allows you to sell medium-risk medical devices or **in vitro diagnostic devices** (**IVDs**).

- Reimbursement rules to the claims that are legitimate. This varies strongly per the insurer, as well as region and country.

- Security and privacy standards including audit frameworks. Think of the **Health Insurance Portability and Accountability Act (HIPAA)**, the **General Data Protection Regulation (GDPR)**, and 510(k).

- Professional standards for clinicians, physicians, nurses, and other care staff.

- Investments by medical companies, including pharmaceutics.

- Innovation – for instance, in automation.

- Legal possibilities to pursue after malpractice.

The important stakeholders in this are the following:

- National as well as local governments such as municipalities.

- Umbrella organizations for care providers, patients, and other groups of interest.

- International institutions such as the **World Health Organization (WHO)**, the **International Standards Organization (ISO)**, and similar regional organizations.

- Vendors and vendor programs. Think of discounts on medical equipment or certain medications.

- Patient groups.

- Unions for professionals to ensure decent wages and working conditions.

- Investors.

- Media in all forms and formats.

All of these formal and informal engagements play a role in the way future healthcare will be organized and they set guardrails and constraints on the architecture of healthcare systems. They make architecture and governance in healthcare extremely complex, especially since there are huge differences per continent, region, and even within regions, countries, or states.

If we want to disrupt this complex system, start focusing on the well-being of the patient, and lower healthcare costs, then we need to look at different systems for organizing healthcare in the future. It calls for the integration of value streams and interoperability between systems. We have to combine the disciplines of systems engineering and community building.

So to recap, complexity is about the (un)predictability of the many possible interactions between all actors within the healthcare system – interactions that can relate to communication about or the intent of the coordination, control, or command of activities. These can be activities in ad-hoc groups or organized in collaborations, such as alliances or corporations to let people direct their health; activities performed in systems or components performing functions such as diagnostics and interventions such as providing treatments and observations; activities that can be classified into case management, stepped care, integrated care, or directed care; activities with ever-increasing interaction that have to adhere to policies and regulations.

We will further discuss embracing this complexity in the following sections of this chapter and make a start by defining DevOps4Care.

Understanding the value of care with DevOps principles

The commonly used definition of DevOps is a set of practices that combines **development** (**dev**) and **operations** (**ops**), typically referring to software development. The goal is to shorten the development life cycle of digital products, whilst maintaining high quality by integrating continuous feedback from the end users.

The most essential rules are listed as follows:

- **Customer-centric action**: Solutions and products are developed with the customer in mind – not only in mind but in some form of co-creation with the customer and users.

- **Create with the end result in mind**: What will a solution do or what will a product look like when it's completely finished? How will it be experienced?

- **Continuous improvement**: A solution or a product is not a one-off thing but must be improved in every iteration.

The DevOps processes and how these are integrated into a continuous cycle are shown in the following diagram:

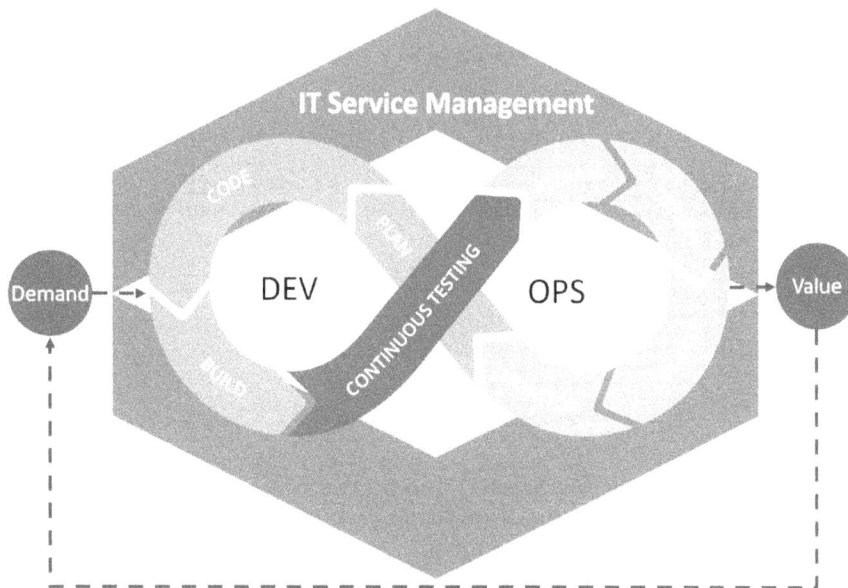

Figure 3.1 – The DevOps cycle

DevOps is widely adopted in IT service management and software development. It helps improve solutions through a continuous loopback into the demands that are set for solutions. Products and services are constantly improved by listening to the customer, retrieving their feedback, and integrating that into the specifications of the product or service. The next release will have improved in quality or include new features, delivering more value to the customers. Modern companies can have multiple releases per day.

An important learning curve in DevOps is that these processes will not work if the development and operations of solutions are siloed. This is a huge problem in healthcare – the industry as a whole and healthcare institutes themselves are heavily siloed. DevOps is all about teams developing and even executing solutions with end-to-end responsibility. These teams work cross-functionally and autonomously, meaning that they can and must take decisions by themselves.

How would that work in the delivery of care? Would DevOps be suitable for the delivery of healthcare? For sure it would mean a disruptive model of delivery, but as we have seen in *Chapter 2, Exploring Relevant Technologies for Healthcare,* with the example of the Danish Naerkliniken, it's certainly not impossible if teams are supported with the right tools and the right skills. Care teams must become multi-disciplinary and qualified for digital work.

The key in DevOps is that it's customer-centric, or in the case of DevOps4Care, patient-centric. It's about delivering value to the patient. **Value, Objectives, Indicators, Confidence, and Experience** (**VOICE**) is a model that incorporates this principle very well. The VOICE model is shown in the following diagram:

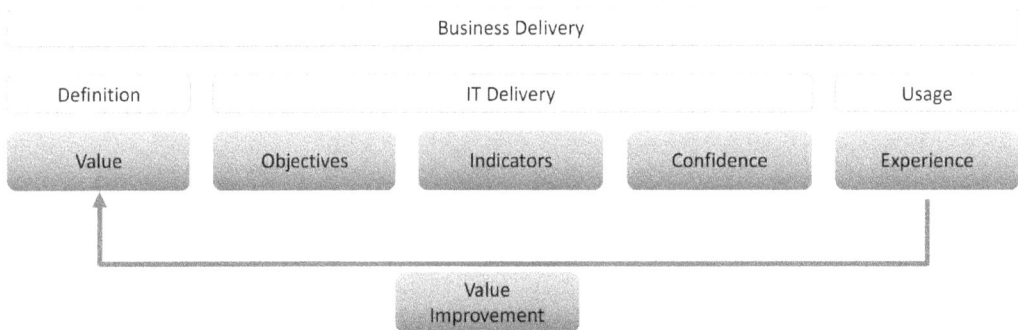

Figure 3.2 – The VOICE model

VOICE was developed by the IT company **Sogeti**. The idea is that value sets the objectives for a product or a service. The objectives are measured by defined indicators. Confidence is about confirming that the value is delivered by achieving the objectives. Experience proves that a product or a service is fulfilling the demands of the business – this is a continuous feedback loop to constantly improve the product or service and add more value to the customer.

If we replace *IT delivery* with *healthcare provisioning* in VOICE, then it almost immediately shows that these models can be used in healthcare too. The business delivery means the output of health, the outcome of lifestyle, and the outlook to participate.

If we combine DevOps with VOICE, we get the following diagram:

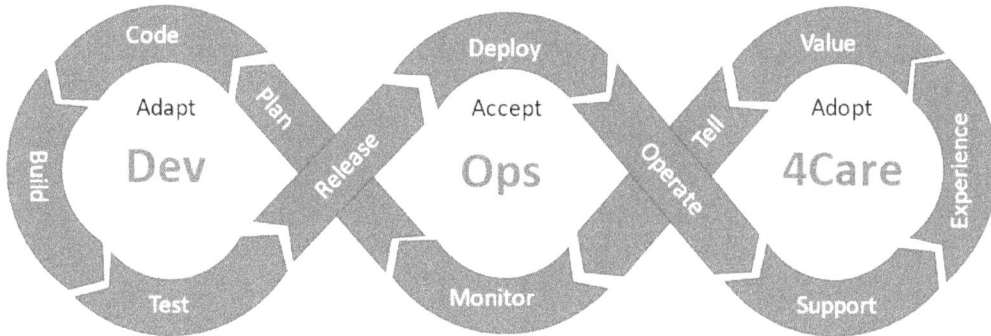

Figure 3.3 – Integrated development, operations, and (health)care: DevOps4Care

The extension *4Care* consists of the *support* to get the confidence to use digital care, *experience* it, *value* it, and be able to *tell* what value improvements need to be defined in the next cycle.

Supporting healthcare activities

Support is usually achieved with a service desk, training sessions when a new system is introduced, and peer support by colleagues who know how to use the systems involved in healthcare activities. We will address this topic in later chapters on how to strengthen this support with actual healthcare workers to create a better experience.

Experiencing healthcare activities

It's during the interactions that take place within healthcare activities where the systems are experienced. This is implicit, but we will see that where the moment of truth happens. Designing and improving how these interactions are experienced is what we will concentrate on as the foundation of transformation. This is explained in further detail in upcoming chapters.

Valuing the healthcare activities

Value is a broad term and very subjective. Understanding value in light of the complexity of experience is the key to translating it into explicit terms that can form a narrative. See the *Defining value in healthcare* section for the terms used to give this narrative structure and meaning.

Telling about the healthcare activities

To close the 4Care feedback loop in DevOps, the storytelling must be taken care of. The value put into a structured narrative via stories feeds the monitoring. Storytelling and exploring these stories will be elaborated on in the next two chapters.

DevOps4Care is all about giving the patients and caregivers a voice to tell the stories that match the different stages in DevOps4Care and bringing change into practice with a **triple-A** rating: **Adapt**, **Accept**, and **Adopt**.

But we need a clear definition of what value is. It's not as simple as a business case. The problem with defining value as a positive outcome of a business case is that organizations tend to start tweaking the financial levers – for example, with cost-cutting. By doing that, we're not adding value to our end customer. In our case, the person wants treatment to improve their health and lifestyle and be able to participate in society. We need to integrate the business case and value creation with a broader perspective.

In the next section, we will discuss what value is in our proposition for healthcare.

Defining value in healthcare

Let's define what value means in healthcare. We will explore this step by step. The steps are shown in the following diagram, including the guardrails of cost, safety, and privacy next to the value itself:

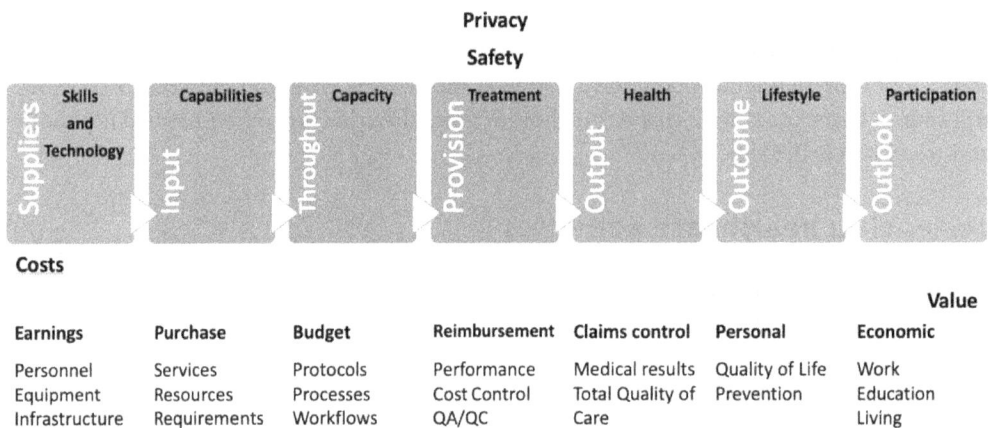

Figure 3.4 – Value creation staging in healthcare

The first stage – on the far-left-hand side of the diagram – is the supply orientation with qualified personnel, equipment, infrastructure, or services. Here, value refers to the wages of personnel and revenue for suppliers. Basically, here, value is about the earnings, as it says at the bottom of the box.

The next stage is input-oriented – the capabilities have to be built by purchasing services and resources in accordance with the requirements.

The preceding stage is followed by throughput, which is process-oriented and focuses on enough delivery capacity, with the protocols and processes made into workflows for the care activities. Care providers have typical departmental budgets for the capacity needed to perform their work. This results in the provisioning of treatments with performance and cost control defined by quality standard parameters. For the work they have done with satisfactory performance, the care providers are reimbursed, in most cases, by insurance companies or public institutions.

So far, this is the traditional way of delivering care. At most, a few care providers are involved with referrals in the chain or clinical pathway. However, we have still no guarantee that we are creating the optimum value for the patient. We are treating one medical problem or health condition and following the protocols. These protocols are, of course, based on proven medical research and clinical claims to ensure the quality of care. However, there is room for greater value in terms of quality of life.

Next, we will be focusing on value in the following three stages – output of health, outcome on lifestyle, and outlook to participate. In these stages, we create value beyond a single care provider or simple referrals in a chain. We aim for the quality of health, life, and eventually participation as the metric of real value. But why is it so difficult to get to these stages of value creation? The answer to that question is a bit cynical – follow the money and you will understand the basic behavior of the stakeholders.

To be fair, the earnings, reimbursement, and economic value stages are typically more tangible than the in-between stages. With that in mind, the *buying power* of teams and departmental budgets are defined within organizations and as part of the value streams. However, for the last three steps (output, outcome, and outlook), it is much harder to create these value streams. Output, outcome, and outlook are less tangible than earnings, reimbursements, and economics. Business cases are much harder to realize in practice to create value streams for these last three stages. Let's explore the cause of that.

Medical protocols treat specific problems and often do not take the outputs of other care activities into account, leading to a disconnect between the output and outcome. The output doesn't take the health experience of an individual patient into consideration very much, other than measuring customer satisfaction after treatment. Medical output, therefore, doesn't generate the full potential value for the patient. However, social care can be more focused on solutions for the patient.

Hence, we can find a solution to create an integrated output for value streams to get to an optimized outcome or outlook. One reason why it can be hard to achieve this is solidarity through insurance. This sounds strange, but insurance creates a disconnect between care usage and care costs. It's different from personal care, such as a fitness club membership. You are willing to pay for a subscription if it improves your health experience. Also, for an employer, there is a more direct relation in terms of care costs, as far as healthy employees take less sick leave. Regardless, we can see that insurance companies have an interest in reducing claims. And last but not least, there is extra economical value coming from a healthier population. Broken value streams can therefore inhibit value creation. In *Chapter 6*, *Applying the Panarchy Principles*, we will learn about some ways to detect these inhibition points and deal with them.

Theoretical insights on this can be found in Michael Porter's **Value-Based HealthCare** (**VBHC**) approach. One important insight from that is that technology is a great enabler in creating this value. This certainly agrees with our experience that creating value streams can only be done through measuring results by collecting data.

This is the real transition in healthcare – relevant data must be collected to determine the value and how to control the value streams – exactly what VOICE aims to achieve. Let's consider bringing DevOps4Care into practice.

One big challenge in creating value lies in enabling disciplines to communicate with each other about value – we need interoperability between systems to enable integration and synchronization through optimized workflows that aim for more individual, personalized healthcare provisioning. To add to the described complexity, we can do this continuously over the whole lifetime of a person. That means we must train care providers in the use of these systems. With that being said, we return to the need for new, digital skills on the part of these providers. Our TiSH has now really begun.

With value better defined, we can understand the complex relations, attitudes, and decisions taken better. Now, we can take this into consideration during the DevOps process. Following value, better designs can be made for the enabling systems.

In the next section, we will take a closer look at the interoperability of systems and discover how we can create an integrated SoS. However, we will learn that it's not so much a matter of getting technology in place. We must address governance in the transformation of healthcare.

Understanding technology in complex systems

Healthcare is, almost by default, not delivered through integrated systems because of different policies and regulations and the variety of technologies. That variety and the lack of integration slows down innovation and transformation in healthcare. How do we change that? This is where the rationale behind the SoS concept becomes relevant to use in the platform that we want to develop as part of our transformation. In other words, to address the complexity of various systems, we need to understand the interoperability of these systems.

Integrating systems or components means that they must connect where they're supposed to. Think of Lego© blocks put together. The blocks are interoperable. The blocks fit together by design. Being able to integrate systems around people needing health attention requires paying the same attention to interoperability.

Interoperability often refers to the ability of computer systems or software to exchange and make use of information that is stored and processed in different systems. Although this definition pertains to computer systems and software, it's applicable to all systems. How do we get the systems and the professionals working with these systems to make use of information across systems in and outside their own organization and provide integrated care?

Technical architects will immediately start thinking of communication protocols, which is a logical thing to do. We have defined these protocols in healthcare systems with, for example, **Health Level Seven (HL7)** as a global standard for securely exchanging healthcare data, **Fast Healthcare Interoperability Resources (FHIR)** as a standard for interoperability, and **Digital Imaging and Communications in Medicine (DICOM)**, which defines the standards for medical images from, for example, CT and MR scanners.

However, the challenge is not so much on the technology side of things – it's more a matter of proper governance and community building to provide that governance.

The more complex the platform becomes, the more governance from the community is required. If we want to understand the real complexity of integrated healthcare, we first need to classify the complexity of the platform and match it with the characteristics of networked care, as defined in *Figure 3.1*.

For this classification, we refer to **System of Systems Engineering (SoSE)** this time. In the following figure, on the left-hand side, the system complexity is classified, and on the right-hand side, we have the associated type of networked care:

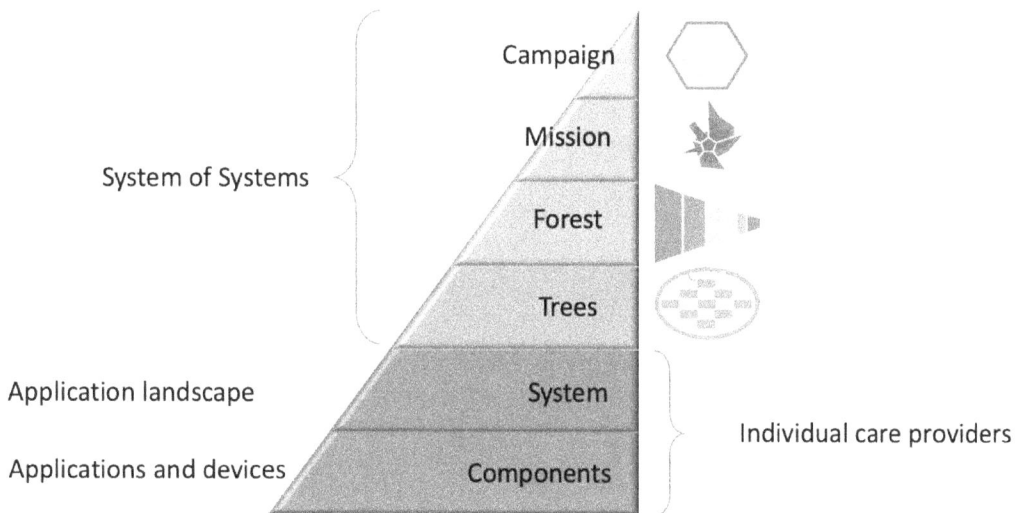

Figure 3.5 – Structuring governance in healthcare systems (adapted from Raymond Deiotte)

Again, we draw some insights from the defense sector. Here, complex systems are very common. As with the rules of engagement for a military campaign, we can imagine the campaign and missions from the ministry or city council formed so that a population with a healthy lifestyle can participate in society. Let's see what we get if we can apply this understanding to TiSH.

At the bottom of the pyramid, we find the components are the resources of individual care providers. These components comprise the traditional applications for processing patient records, picture archiving from CT scans, HR and logistics applications, and also e-health devices or other resources such as sensors that define some kind of health condition. At this level, application components are usually not integrated – they mostly deliver input from single observations or perform single tasks. For care provisioning, the components in the application landscape are integrated via processes and workflows as provided by ERP applications. This is the system on an organizational level.

To get an integrated view of the overall condition of the patient, in networked care case management, we need to get these systems and components to work with other health care providers first. Their own systems will branch out, communicating with the systems of these other providers to communicate about each other's activities. This is called a **Trees-level SoS**.

The collaboration in stepped care, enabling care professionals to orientate on possible (clinical) pathways, requires the Trees-level SoS of the care providers to agree on the coordination of activities in this collaboration and form a **Forest-level SoS**.

Next is the cooperation in integrated care where all the components of all the organizations combine to act as a single **Mission-level SoS**, control the concurrent care activities of all involved in the care network, and acknowledge the effects of these activities.

To get to the desired outcome for individuals and the population at large in directed care, joint decision-making and integrated workflows are required at the Campaign-level to realize the goal for the patient and population to participate in social environments again – as in, the outlook value. This calls for directing and commanding, which is at the top of the pyramid – defining the joint missions, deciding how to fulfill those missions, and acting upon them by population management.

> **Tip**
>
> The detailed, scientific article which *Figure 3.5* is based on, *A Novel Approach to Mission-Level Engineering of Complex Systems of Systems; Addressing Integration and Interoperability Shortfalls by Interrogating the Interstitials*, by *Ray Deiotte* (ISSAC Corp) and *Robert K. Garrett, Jr* (Missile Defense Agency), is also a good starting point for modeling a digital twin for healthcare provisioning and defining the requirements of the technology to develop. It's very comprehensive, but demonstrates what complex systems are can how they can be modeled.

The takeaway from this article is the term *"interstitials,"* which is used to define the importance of paying attention to designing the connections between constituent systems. That's why we are going to focus on **Interoperability and Integration** (**I & I**) for each tread of the TiSH staircase. But that's a topic for *Chapter 8, Learning How Interaction Works in Technology-Enabled Care Teams*.

Now is the time to remember the value creation stages that we studied in *Figure 3.3* about value creation staging in healthcare; remember the stages developing from earnings to the output, outcome, and outlook. If we were to combine the horizontal value creation stages with the vertical complexity hierarchy that we showed in *Figure 3.5*, you can probably already guess that there is a correlation between the value and the complexity, as can be seen in the following diagram:

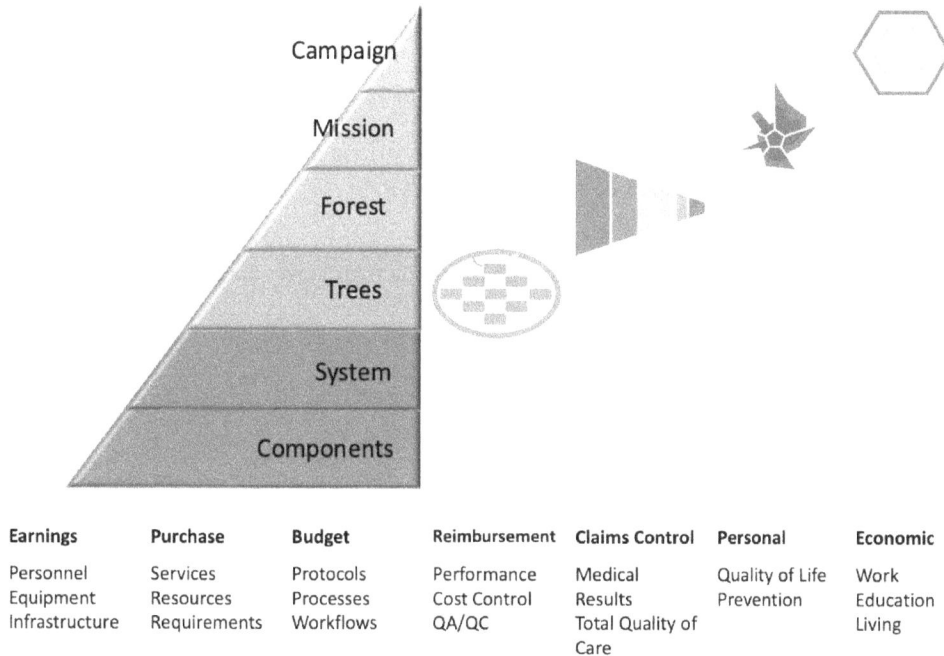

Earnings	Purchase	Budget	Reimbursement	Claims Control	Personal	Economic
Personnel	Services	Protocols	Performance	Medical	Quality of Life	Work
Equipment	Resources	Processes	Cost Control	Results	Prevention	Education
Infrastructure	Requirements	Workflows	QA/QC	Total Quality of Care		Living

Figure 3.6 – Complexity versus value stages

With proper governance in place, we can define the standards for integrated systems in terms of Mission Level-SoSE. Major tech companies and their capabilities will play a significant role in this because it is too complex for any care provider. We will explore their role in the final section of this chapter.

Understanding the role of major technology providers

Technology providers are enablers – with the technology that these companies develop, they can support medical staff and patients. We have seen in the previous section that the existence of technical protocols such as FHIR and DICOM doesn't solve the challenges of I & I by themselves. Technology is not a magic wand.

However, we are seeing the role of these providers grow and they are having more impact. With an in-depth understanding of clinical processes, they develop technology that professionals and patients can use intuitively for medical purposes.

There's a major shift happening. Technology providers are no longer just an enabler. They are transforming into drivers of innovation as well as transformation. How did this evolve? To start with, money plays a huge role in this. Innovation means investing and that's what these technology companies can do. These firms simply have deep pockets. Innovations are their lifeline.

Secondly, they know *how* to develop innovations. That's because they have that required mindset. A lot of these companies are not hindered by regulations and policies from the start. They can start from a blank sheet, develop a solution, and along the way, iterate and improve the solution as issues occur. They don't start with the roadblocks of regulations and policies. They start with the end goal in mind – the health and well-being of a patient.

Lastly, most of these companies have adopted DevOps as a working methodology to speed up their development and get constant feedback on products and services.

Let's explore what's needed for an Mission Level-SoS interoperable healthcare proposition required for harmonizing the outcome or outlook value. The following figure gives an a priori solution with all the recognizable elements we have covered:

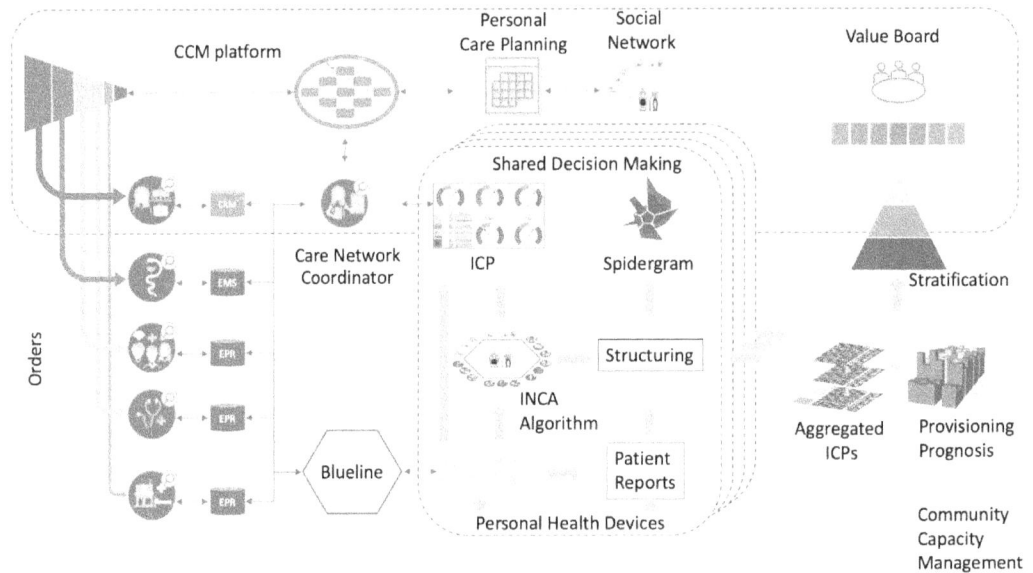

Figure 3.7 – An a priori solution for sustainable health(care)

In the middle, we have the INCA algorithm to optimize the personal hexagon where all care is centered around the patient. This is translated into an **Individual Care Plan** (**ICP**) projected with a **Community Capacity Management** (**CCM**) platform on a Naerklinikken-style **EHealthCare Model** (**ECM**) on the left, providing care per problem or condition. On the right-hand side, information is gathered to simulate the projected type and capacity to serve the population in the community in the near future. This is used by the value board to make decisions on investments and contract the required capacity with the help of the value creation stages.

It seems deceptively easy to realize, but we will see that convincing all the stakeholders at the same time takes time. We will also see that value creation staging will help.

An important question is – why should big tech invest in this? It is common sense that technology can enable transformation. Once the first examples and evidence are delivered through initiatives such as Amazon Care, Buurtzorg, Nearklinikken, and INCA, it will attract investors. Note that Amazon Care started with its own employees and their families as the community. So, they could act as the value board deciding for themselves with closed-loop value streams – one of the success factors.

Big tech can speed up transformation by making sure the opportunities they pursue are interoperable and can be integrated into the relevant care platforms, as in the following examples:

- On the infrastructure level, the cloud services of Microsoft, AWS, and Google can be used for rapid scaling. Kubernetes-based architectures with containers and container orchestration can help with interoperability here.

- Amazon as a customer-focused logistics company can facilitate the generic process of providing the right health devices, services, and medicine at the point of care when it is needed. No special healthcare knowledge is required for such operations.

- Others such as Apple and Samsung offer very good services on personal devices including vital signs, activity tracking, and personal security. They offer app builders and accessory vendors a safe platform. However, to date, they often do not yet integrate into a seamlessly integrated personal health environment. There are examples of patients with Type 2 diabetes using eighteen apps without the ability to merge all their data into a meaningful dashboard.

- On the professional side, companies such as GE, Philips, and Siemens Healthineers, with long traditions in medicine, can and are developing more and more clinical diagnostics to use in local practices and as wearables, making it possible to shift healthcare to the left in the Nearklinikken ECM model.

Together, these companies can and should create innovative design spaces for SMEs to enable them to come up with new solutions – be they medication dispensers, social robots, home automation, or, one of our personal favorites, a hip airbag to give people with mobility problems more confidence and cushion their hip if they fall, preventing medical care. This hip airbag was an instant hit on increasing outlook value and direct contribution to participation at low cost.

Summary

This chapter served as an introduction to the methodologies that we will explore in more detail over the course of this book. These methodologies form the foundation of DevOps4Care and TiSH. We unpacked the complexity of the transformation by studying the policies and regulations that form the guardrails for provisioning healthcare first. We then discussed how we could transform healthcare by using DevOps principles. We learned that DevOps starts with the demands – the voice of the customer – and tries to translate these demands into specifications for products and services, including continuous feedback. These principles are also applicable to healthcare services. We also saw that we need different skills in healthcare to start this transformation.

The most important lesson is that we can use DevOps and other methods to start creating real value for the patient. The key is the integration of care value streams, as opposed to acting on addressing one specific medical condition, as with most contemporary healthcare. With integrated care, focusing on the overall health experience of the patient, we will create new value. Combined outputs create the outlook value – enabling the patient to participate in their communities again. Care is no longer provided in separate care episodes per condition (or siloed), but all conditions are integrated into one care program.

We concluded that integration and interoperability between systems are the key to achieving the goal of enabling the outlook of participation. This adds immense complexity to the solution, requiring an understanding of SoSE in the transformation task force to address these challenges. With that in mind, we constructed an a priori solution for sustainable healthcare, incorporating best practices from Amazon Care, Buurtzorg, Nearklinikken, and INCA. Finally, we discussed the role of big tech to enable the realization of such a solution.

This chapter was more about the methodology to correlate and validate value with stakeholders in networked care. In the next chapter, we will zoom in on the skills of the professionals in care and learn more about human interaction in the new delivery models.

Further reading

- *Enterprise DevOps for Architects* by Jeroen Mulder, Packt Publishing, 2021
- *Quality for DevOps Teams* by Rik Marselis, Berend van Veenendaal, Dennis Geurts and Wouter Ruigrok, Sogeti, 2020
- *The DevOps Career Handbook* by John Knight and Nate Swenson, Packt Publishing, 2022
- *Healthcare Digital Transformation* by Edward W. Marx and Paddy Padmanabhan, CRC Press, 2021
- *Redefining Health Care: Creating Value-Based Competition on Results*, by Micheal E. Porter and Elizabeth Olmsted Teisberg
- *A Novel Approach to Mission-Level Engineering of Complex Systems of Systems; Addressing Integration and Interoperability Shortfalls by Interrogating the Interstitials*, by Ray Deiotte (ISSAC Corp) and Robert K. Garrett, Jr (Missile Defense Agency)

4
Including the Human Factor in Transformation

Learning in a group will accelerate understanding. Indeed MoM TiSH sends us to school and interacts with the others in the classroom.

In the previous chapter, we introduced the complexity of healthcare when it comes to the transformation into data-driven healthcare. However, we also promised to keep a hundred percent focus on the persons working on their or someone else's health. How do we take human factors into consideration? What skills do care providers need in the ongoing digitalization of healthcare?

The theme for this chapter is viewpoints on **human measure**. Our transformation taskforce, including the system engineering architects and community builders in healthcare, will apply one golden rule to achieve this: it's always about the patient and the people who care for them. Healthcare is about humans. How do we make sure that humans—patients, but also next of kin, social workers, and medical staff—don't get lost in the regulations, systems, and technology of the platform we build? How do we prevent them from getting lost in data? And how do we balance between man and machine? All these are relevant questions that we will try to answer in this chapter.

In this chapter, we're going to cover the following main topics:

- Introducing human-centric **information technology (IT)**
- Human interaction on the health journey
- Working together in **technology-enabled care (TEC)** teams
- Defining a new way of organizing healthcare

Introducing human-centric IT

In the previous chapter, we stated that digital transformation requires new disciplines. We introduced **systems engineering** (**SE**) and community building as skills for our transformation taskforce team. But what about the digital and other skills of the personnel within the care organizations and other stakeholders? In this chapter, we will eventually conclude that we need new roles in healthcare to get the transformation executed in practice. An **e-nurse**—to put it simply, a nurse with specific digital skills—is such a role. But also remember the **e-doctor** from the *Nearklinikken*. We will come to speak about this later in this chapter from both an engineering approach and a community-building approach.

Starting with engineering, let's get back to the basic principles of **development-operations** (**DevOps**). Companies that adopt DevOps work with autonomous tools that are **end-to-end** (**E2E**) responsible for the development and operations of a product or a service. Could we plot that model to healthcare? The short and obvious answer is *yes*. But we need to get a deeper understanding first of the value streams and dynamics in healthcare and what these mean for the roles and tasks that are required in this domain.

The goal that we are trying to achieve is to increase the value for the patient. We want to create real value for the patient by integrating workstreams aimed at the outlook, which is participation. To recap the learning from the previous chapter, outlook leading to participation means that a patient can—for instance—get back to work or participate in a social life again. That is the goal of care, and not just treating a specific condition.

As explained in the last chapter with DevOps4Care, we added *support*, *experience*, *value*, and *tell* features to the feedback loop to iterate to the desired value creation. Value is created in experienced interactions.

Increasing value means more and more data streams to be developed and operated. What does this mean for the activities of involved personnel, patients, and persons in other roles alike in the *4Care* part of DevOps4Care? What is their perspective? Let's find out.

Including 4Care in DevOps

DevOps is all about keeping in touch with the users: Is the platform user-friendly? Is it performing well? Is it making my work as a professional easier? Therefore, users need to be involved in the DevOps process. When we start implementing DevOps4Care, one of the first things that we need to do is to position the user well in the organization and empower them. We will learn how that will look when we study the new role of **storytellers** in healthcare. It's giving the healthcare professional the opportunity to have regular talks and conversations with the back offices to express their concerns and experiences with the systems in detail. A simple "does not work" is a start, but something such as "filling in that form takes me a lot of time and I don't understand why I have to fill it completely" is already better. The storyteller is a pivotal role in adopting new technology in care provisioning. They provide feedback for continuous improvement and innovation.

Before we dive into the 4Care component, we need to get a better understanding of DevOps as an overall concept and why it's perfectly usable in healthcare.

To start, we must begin reasoning on experience level. This means that we start with exploring user stories. This is a common approach in DevOps and agile methods. A user story is a short description of what a user wants. Typically, user stories are used as the start of product or software development. A user story consists of a few sentences in the user's common language stating what the user does or must do as part of their job. In our case, a user story should be something a patient or care worker *desires*. In other words: what do the patient and their caregivers want or need? Next, a user story must have a certain format. A typical format for a user story looks like this: *As a {persona}, I want to be able to {action} so that I can {goal}.*

> **Note**
>
> Remember we mentioned earlier that we need to automate DevOps4Care to address the fact that programmers are an even scarcer resource than care personnel? Let's have a small intermezzo to contemplate that before we proceed. Imagine that the preceding story of the persona is enough to make a new app. What are the possibilities to realize code by just telling stories? Hold that thought—we'll come back to it later in this chapter.

From the user story, we can derive and set objectives and requirements. What should a solution aim for, and what requirements do we need to fulfill to achieve the objectives? Even more important, when do we consider a solution to be ready? In development, this is often referred to as the **Definition of Done (DoD)**. The DoD sets a very clear description of the status when a product or a service is ready to be delivered. From that point onward, feedback is retrieved to improve the product or service. We will discover in the next sections how this feedback loop is integrated into models that we can use for the delivery of healthcare, but first, we will study user stories.

Defining user stories

In this section, we turn to the users of the systems. In different stages of DevOps4Care, we involve three types of users as storytellers. We can then plot these storytellers to the different stages in the user story. These triple-A stages are *adapt*, *accept*, and *adopt*. This addresses the adoption of new or modified systems and ways of working by all users. How would that translate into a concrete model with real user stories? We will have the following:

- **Lead users** who help in the development process (*adapt*). These lead users are able to tell or show the developers what the needs are. Lead users are not bound to a role. They can be a patient, next of kin or a friend, or a caregiver. They are highly motivated.

- **Specialized users** who enroll the solutions into the operations (*accept*). We can think of an e-nurse. An e-nurse is a trained nurse with extra skills to understand how new or adapted systems would fit into healthcare provisioning and advise what has to be changed before it can be accepted.

- **Supporting users** who provide peer support (*adopt*) to all other users in understanding the *why* and the *how*. They typically have coaching skills to tell the story to users, operators, and developers alike.

The number of users scales with every stage, from a few lead users to more specialized users and many supporting users. Consequently, a different way to look at this is at what development stage these storyteller types can be the most effective in terms of the following scaling phases: *start-up*, *scale-up*, and *scaler*. Let's look at this in more detail here:

- The initial development of processes and technology adaptation is the *start-up* phase with help of the lead users to guide the process

- *Scale-up* is done through specialized users such as an e-nurse and an e-doctor who have accepted the processes and systems to use in the field

- The supporting users are used as the *scaler*, making sure that processes and systems are adopted on a wide basis in the field

Recognizing these three types of users in the organization makes sure that the stories from these actual users are the input for the development process.

How is this done in practice? Let's have a look at *Figure 4.1*, which is based on the **Activity Theory** and the triangle model developed by Y. Engeström, used for the *Digicoach* training program developed by *Q-Consult Zorg* for the healthcare innovation institute, ZonMw commissioned by the **Dutch Ministry of Public Health, Welfare and Sport (VWS)**.

> Tip
>
> For more insights, the scientific research behind the Activity Theory can be explored. A good starting point is the bundle of articles *Learning and Expanding with Activity Theory*, edited by Annalisa Sannino, Harry Daniels, and Kris D. Gutiérrez at `http://www.cambridge.org/9780521760751` where in part Five, Article 16 of *Who is Acting in an Activity System* by Rita Engeström explores the application of Activity Theory in a healthcare setting.

Remember that in the last chapter, we emphasized interactions and activities are key to the experience. The source of the stories is in these activities and interactions. Therefore, model structuring activities to identify relations to understand the complexity is what we need. That is the Activity Theory and, specifically, the activity triangle. This will help in analyzing the narrative of the stories. Stories are in the center of gravity in the activity triangle shown in the following diagram:

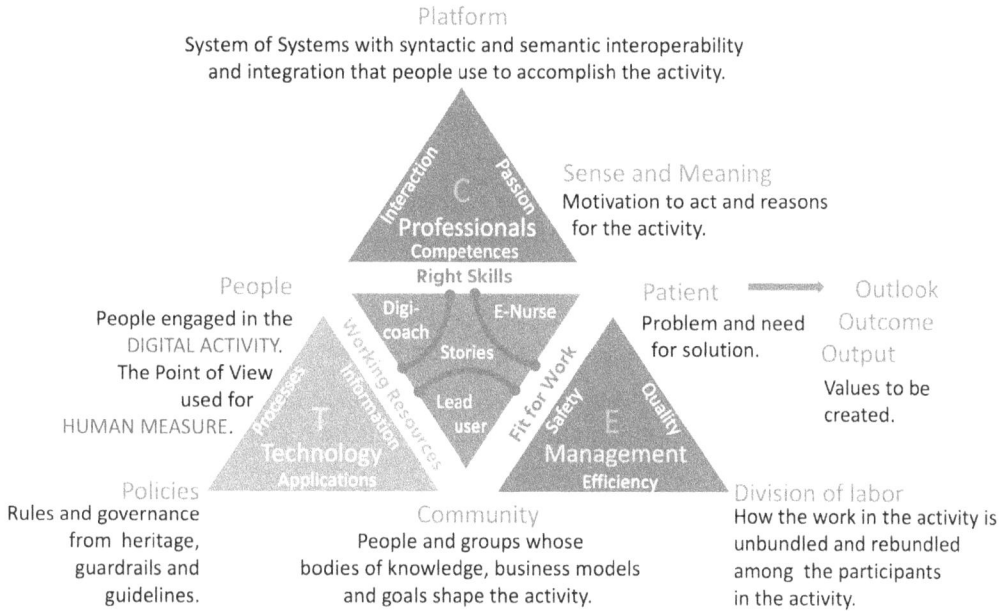

Platform
System of Systems with syntactic and semantic interoperability
and integration that people use to accomplish the activity.

Sense and Meaning
Motivation to act and reasons for the activity.

People
People engaged in the DIGITAL ACTIVITY.
The Point of View used for HUMAN MEASURE.

Patient
Problem and need for solution.

Outlook
Outcome
Output
Values to be created.

Policies
Rules and governance from heritage, guardrails and guidelines.

Community
People and groups whose bodies of knowledge, business models and goals shape the activity.

Division of labor
How the work in the activity is unbundled and rebundled among the participants in the activity.

Figure 4.1 – Digital healthcare activity triangle (Courtesy of Q-Consult Zorg)

The *Digicoach* program was developed to increase the capacity of peer support on the actual work floors where care is provided. Care workers of all sorts were trained to understand digitalization from the point of view of the people engaged in digital activities and learn how to be a coach for their co-workers.

The *activity triangle* relates the care workers engaged in digital activities related to the 30 terms such as *interaction*, *competences*, *information*, and *processes* shown in *Figure 4.1*. The digicoaches (digital coaches) are trained to support their peers on the work floor, and when feedback is needed from management and technology suppliers, they have—from the defined terms—the vocabulary to express themselves. They have learned to tell stories.

Now, we can put this to good use in DevOps4Care. As mentioned shortly before, we added the *support*, *experience*, *value*, and *tell* features to the feedback loop to iterate to the desired value creation.

For each of these features in 4Care, the digicoach can express themself with the activity triangle terms shown in *Figure 4.1*, as follows:

- **Support** is extended by the digicoach for the *right skills*. This form of peer support coexists with the more traditional help or service desk.

- **Experience** of the users is noticed through their acquired coaching skills in the Activity Triangle terms of *policies, division of labor, community*, the *sense and meaning* of it, and the *interaction* characteristics of the *platform*.

- **Value** for the *patient* is understood in terms of problems and solutions for *output* in better health, *outcome* in health lifestyle, and *outlook* on participation.

- **Telling stories** about how the *interaction* with the *platform* used in the working *processes* influences the experience of the users and the value for both users and *patients*.

The digicoach is also trained to be aware of the relations between the other terms of the activity triangle to be better able to indicate problems and room for improvement.

Using these terms in the narrative helps to format the story as input for the developers, like so:

As a {professional doctor}, I want to be able to {interact remotely with the nurse present with the patient} so that I can {inspect the wound} {using the smartglass the nurse is wearing}.

The terms not mentioned are not forgotten but form the explicit context of the story to take into consideration during development.

The same is true for the e-nurse (or e-doctor) specialized user, with the distinction that they are not only aware of the relationships but have a better understanding of them. They are expected to give more structured stories.

The lead user has an intrinsic motivation and direct interest to develop specific applications or improve them. It is quite common for lead users to show the way it can or should be done. To capture their stories, the aforementioned digicoaches and specialized users can conduct a semi-structured interview.

This is how these three roles act as storytellers for the input of DevOps iterations, and they comply with the one rule: it's always about the patient and the people who care for them. Healthcare is about humans.

With the terms in the activity triangle, we have learned that from a viewpoint of people such as professionals engaged in digital activities, it's about interactions between people and platforms—interactions with applications to access information to engage with passion in the activity with the patient, an engagement requiring digital competences based on the right skills. That's what we are going to talk about in the next section.

Human interaction on the health journey

In the activity triangle shown in *Figure 4.1*, we have identified that the relation between the people and the platform is the interaction between them, given the context of the other entities. In daily practice, this translates to many types of applications to support the interactions in which they engage in their activities throughout the health journey of the patient. In *Chapter 1, Understanding (the Need for) Transformation, Figure 1.7*, we depicted the personal health journey with the desired output of better health with meaningful health information needed in interactions.

Complexity is in the number of possible interactions between all types of actors—a number of interactions that, in the reality of healthcare provisioning, very quickly become very complex indeed, certainly within health journeys in networked care. To embrace the complexity, we need to model these interactions from the caregiver's perspective, both within the teams of care professionals and between the teams also providing care for the patient.

The following diagram is a representation of the types of data streams, workflows, and processes for these interactions. You will recognize medical data, planning data, financial data, logistics data, support data, data on **human resources (HR)**, and communications used in activities:

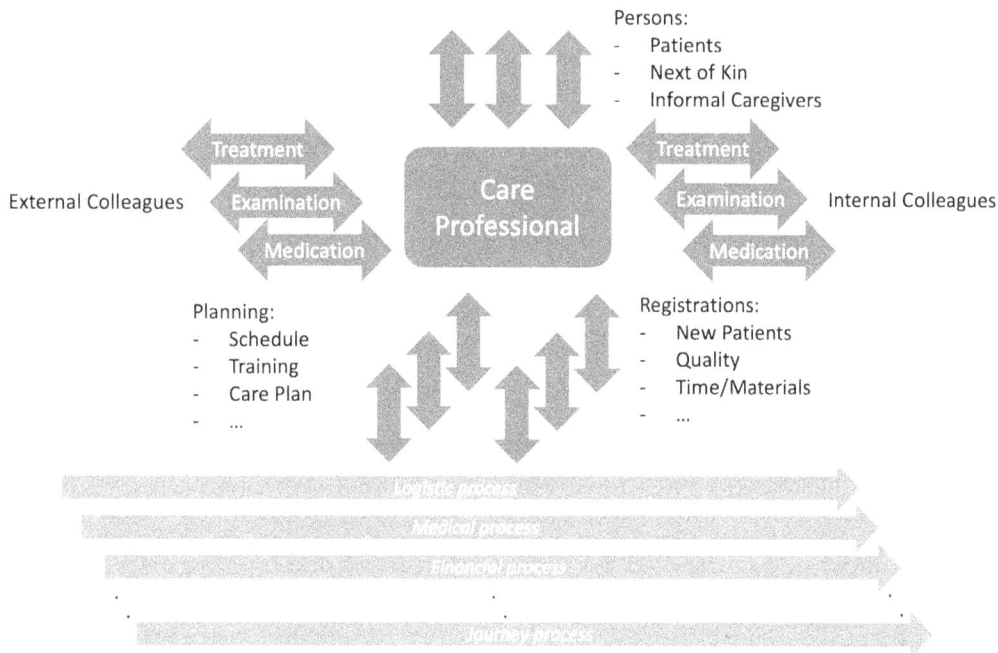

Figure 4.2 – Example of data streams in care provisioning

It's not very hard to see and understand that all these data streams can easily lead to an overload of information for the care provider, who sits in the middle of the diagram, yet all this data is required to enable the interactions to provide care. However, an overload of data can mean that data is not processed into meaningful information to be utilized in decision-making. What is worse is it will distract from personal attention to the patient. This can all lead to undesired effects, such as higher workloads and lower job satisfaction. Gone is the passion—hardly something to keep the sector attractive for professionals. Therefore, traditional automation of processes is no longer improving healthcare; on the contrary, it inhibits progress.

Hence, we must understand what we need to do when it comes to designing and engineering integrated digital care. We must design systems in such a way that users can easily understand and use these systems. This is the field of **Human Systems Integration** (**HSI**). We will learn more about this in the next section.

Working with HSI

Let's have another look at *Figure 4.2* and identify different workflows and processes. We recognize the following processes:

- Registration of patients
- Scheduling of appointments
- Defining the patient journey (**customer relationship management**, or **CRM**)
- Filing discharge instructions
- Initiating reimbursement and payment
- Filing training admissions
- Processing support requests
- Supporting audit procedures

But it's not just the process itself—with every process, we must consider privacy, security, patient safety, and value as well. This will add to the number of interactions within the process and thus more stimuli for the worker, meaning more attention points. Does technology lift the burden of this? Unfortunately, that's often not the case since healthcare has to deal with a lot of legacy systems. Workers must scroll through many fields and fill out various pages in systems, creating an even bigger load. The complaint of having too many administrative tasks in healthcare is an often-heard tune.

This is a bad thing, as you will see in the example of increasing complexity by the increased number of interactions. So, how do we decrease it?

Here's where HSI can help. HSI comes with a comprehensive set of principles that integrate nicely with the principles of DevOps. Some of the principles from the perspective of care workers are set out here:

- Registering only once and reusing data
- Combining actions into one step in the workflow
- Automating as much as possible; also, things such as **single sign-on (SSO)**
- A common look and feel
- Single support desk

Keep in mind that this will apply also to patients, but is more complicated in the last two points. A common look and feel for the patient is very personal and has to do with all interactions, including using apps for travel, banking, shopping, gaming, and much more. A healthcare application must take into consideration that different types of users have different user requirements.

It's a good idea to leverage a bit on what HSI is and how it could benefit design in healthcare systems. To put it simply, HSI encompasses an approach to developing systems that focuses on the interfaces between man and machine. To achieve optimal interaction between humans and technical systems, HSI includes multiple domains, as outlined here:

- Improved utilization of manpower
- Reduced training costs for using technology
- Improved user acceptance
- Decreased life-cycle costs of systems because of decreased need for redesign

HSI is a topic within SE that we introduced as an important discipline to be included in our transformation taskforce. SE is applied in designing complex environments such as aerospace or traffic control where vast amounts of data are used for decision-making. That's why we think it's a good place to look for best practices to be used in healthcare. So, let's have a look.

Recently, a new vision of SE, called **Systems Engineering Vision 2035** (or **Vision 35** for short) was released. In that vision, systems in 2035 will be even more autonomous and more interconnected, and stakeholders will expect these systems to be safe, secure, resilient, and affordable. Obviously, this includes systems for healthcare.

> Tip
>
> The **International Council on Systems Engineering (INCOSE)** offers a huge generic knowledge base to explore, with Vision 35 as an excellent starting point. Have a look at `https://violin-strawberry-9kms.squarespace.com/model-based-practices`.

One of the key elements in Vision 35 is model-based working. INCOSE states the future of SE is predominantly model-based. Vision 35 implies the use of virtual, digital twin-based models that can be reused many times and that enable a high degree of collaboration. To put this in a more comprehensive wording, virtual models allow for intensive user testing and reduce the costs of engineering dramatically. Cloud and cloud-native technologies with high-capacity compute infrastructure are preferred in future engineering.

The challenge is that the many legacy systems in place within healthcare prevent an ideal design for systems that comply with the HSI principles. Legacy systems are often based on 30-year-old design principles and are typically monolithic, whereas in modern system design, services are designed as microservices, using cloud and cloud-native technology. Let's look at this in a bit more detail here:

- **Monolithic**: Systems designed as one piece. Typically, these systems are capable of handling multiple tasks, but components in the systems are tightly coupled. Changing the architecture is complex.

- **Microservices**: Systems built as microservices consist of loosely coupled, independent services that have been developed and deployed separately. These independent services can integrate with other services using **application programming interfaces** (**APIs**). These systems are more flexible and scalable. Changes to these systems are easier since updates and upgrades can be executed per service instead of for the entire system, but require more governance on integration.

If we design according to microservices architectures, the integration of systems becomes more manageable. The driver for this, however, is not technology itself but to relieve the burden on staff. A way to do that is to create interoperability between systems and—especially—data streams so that staff get the exact right data at the right place and time. Interoperability requires that we design with integration in mind—integration of data streams, processes, and workflows.

HSI can have several stages to integrate, as outlined here:

- **Screen integration**: Bigger screens with more room to display the **user interfaces** (**UIs**) of different systems and the ability to cut and paste. Not ideal, but the first step for task integration by the user, assisted with the presentation level.

- **Robotic process automation** (**RPA**) to automate processes. Suitable for simple rule-based administration tasks and point-of-care process automation assisted by **artificial intelligence** (**AI**).

- Integration of workflow engines such as Zapier and **If This Then That** (**IFTTT**) and integration platforms from leading **enterprise resource planning** (**ERP**)/CRM and **electronic patient record** (**EPR**) solution providers for integration on a workflow level.

- HSI first-principle redesign (sometimes referred to as brownfield or refactoring) to address all levels at once.

- A new modern HSI system taking fully into account all new developments in the automation of DevOps4Care. We asked a question to imagine how storytelling can drive development directly. We can think of using, for example, **Azure Generative Pretrained Transformer 3 (Azure GPT-3)** to generate code based on the narrative from the stories. We think this is, in the end, needed for a large-scale transformation.

Building **greenfield** is one solution to leapfrog HSI, meaning that we build new systems, according to the HSI principles, from the ground up. This is one of the common transformation strategies. We would build a new healthcare network and transfer services and involved personas—stakeholders, providers, patients—one by one. However, we must still deal with the legacy systems that are hard to replace or rebuild without disrupting critical-care processes in a dramatic way. But what we can do is build an interaction model alongside the patient's journey as a starting point, focusing on the interaction between humans and systems, and limiting the number of interactions that users must have with underlying systems. We can build greenfield cockpits and dashboards as tools for interaction. We can also automate processes.

Designing human interaction

For those interested in the *how*, a discipline that excels in supporting interactions is the design of UIs in these cockpits and dashboards. Without exaggerating, this is, in our experience, by far the biggest success factor for successful digital transformation. Comprehensive UIs are essential for an optimal **user experience** (**UX**). It's the *crux*, so to speak. To make this more tangible, we can think of a UI as the comprehensive, transparent entrance to underlying systems.

A UI is the first level of interaction between humans and systems. In architecture, UIs are commonly referred to as **systems of engagement** (**SOEs**), whereas the underlying systems that hold and process the data are referred to as **systems of record** (**SORs**). Humans engage in activities through SOEs, so these must be extremely user-friendly.

The number of interactions in the engagement layer should be limited to patterns that can lead to direct actions—only those with a direct impact on the activities influencing the health condition of the patient for the better. Obviously, the technology guiding the care provider in understanding the interactions, identifying relevant issues, and taking the right, highest-priority decisions must be user-friendly.

With this, we concluded the first tread of **Transformation into Sustainable Healthcare** (**TiSH**) for people skilled in digital activities for TEC. Next, we'll talk about interaction in TEC teams.

Working together in TEC teams

In the previous section, we concluded that we needed to build new systems. Think of SOEs, such as the cockpits and dashboards in aerospace that limit the number of actions that users have to execute and avoid an information overload. Once properly designed, these newly designed systems form a basis to work together with other team members, and if all team members can utilize technology, then we have a TEC team. This will also have an effect on supporting systems.

The different types of storytellers in the team are trained in listening to the users and are able to tell the story to the enabling management and developers of technology. The storytellers must be able to use certain words and concepts in their narrative to be understood. They have learned to use the terms of the activity triangle, but those terms have to be detailed. Although people are not strict, digital transformation requires specific definitions, such as for processes. This is shown in the following diagram, where a simple model is plotted to the required processes:

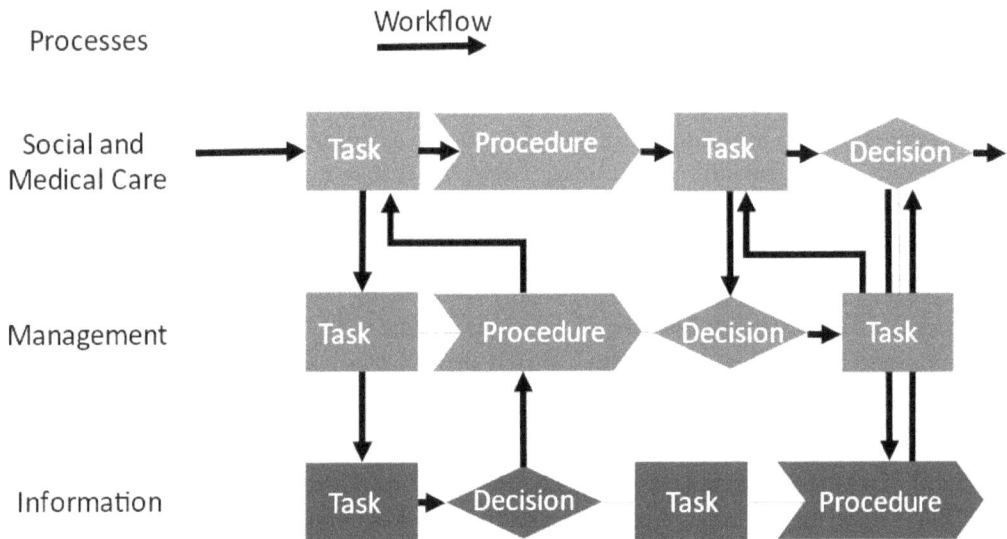

Figure 4.3 – Representation of workflows and processes

The technology layer, where information—data—is processed and systems are built and used, is depicted at the bottom of the diagram. The enabling management layer sits in the middle, whereas the top layer is the actual care layer or the layer where the TEC team operates, interacts, and provides care.

Provisioning is carried out in activities that consist of the following:

- **Actions**: Discrete activities performed by stakeholders or automated in a system
- **Tasks**: Series of related actions taken to achieve specified results or outcomes
- **Procedures**: Sequential tasks that form a distinct phase of a workflow (or protocol if it is regulated)

- **Processes**: Activities that contribute toward achieving larger goals or objectives, such as medical, management, and communication objectives

- **Workflows**: Series of actions, tasks, and procedures over the processes performed to achieve a set output by an actor

We have now defined a process model for telling stories for lean digitization with only relevant interactions for the people engaged in the activities and creating skills needed for digital transformation. This will shape and guide teams to work in a data-driven way, but always with a strong human focus.

> Tip
>
> Note that what we discussed is oversimplified. The reality is much more complex. To get a good appreciation of it, we refer to the **International Organization for Standardization (ISO)** *13940*, of which a visualization can be found on the website `http://www.contsys.org`. A link is given in the *Further reading* section at the end of the chapter.

The green triangle in the middle of the diagram in *Figure 4.1* is also representing the three roles in the TEC team for this. The TEC team incorporates digitally proficient professionals, uses technology, and is embedded in the management of an organization as a change agent. It is the leading example for the rest of the organization. From this position, it helps other **professionals**, works with **management** on continuous improvements, and voices stories to **technology** providers inside and outside the organization, all with the purpose of creating a voice telling stories matching the different stages in DevOps4Care and bringing change into practice with a **triple-A** rating: *adapt, accept, adopt.*

Now that we have activities in a sequence or workflow with processes and tasks, it's time to decide in what order they have to be carried out on the health journey—how to decide on the right things in the right way at the right pace.

Data-driven decisions with OODA

In the previous sections, we introduced DevOps4Care and TEC teams. We learned that in the current system landscape in healthcare, there's a high risk of information overload. Hence, we explored frameworks that enable us to build new systems that limit the number of interactions between professionals and systems and avoid the overload of data. However, teams do need data. The systems that we design, build, and operate should enable professionals to get the right data at the right place and right moment. They need the data to take decisions on the health journey. We can be inspired by how customer journeys are supported in general with the interaction of **touchpoints** and **moments of truth** in *Chapter 8, Learning How Interaction Works in Technology-Enabled Care Teams*, where we will address this in more detail. For now, it's important to know that decisions have to be made. We need the TEC teams to become data-driven to do that.

What does *data-driven* mean? It means that organizations or humans take decisions based on data as evidence and not only on experiences or intuition. Doesn't experience play a role at all? On the contrary. Working data-driven is, above all, working based on facts. These facts are collected from data that is analyzed with analytics tools. These tools translate data, using data models, into meaningful and useful information. The information combined with knowledge and—indeed—experience form insights. Insights are input for decisions and actions.

This is a recurring theme in all types of decisions. Therefore, we can use the **Observe, Orient, Decide, Act (OODA)** loop developed by the American military strategist and air force colonel John Boyd to visualize this recurring process, as follows:

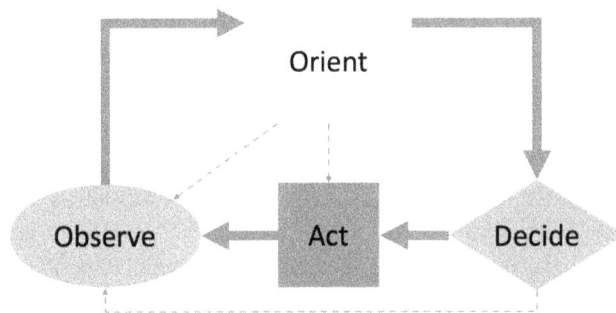

Figure 4.4 – Basic OODA model

It's a simple but very powerful model that will help us greatly in embracing the complexity, as we will see in the remainder of this book.

In the acronym **OODA, Observe** means gathering data and facts, **Orient** for using it to make information on which we can **Decide** to **Act**. That is the main loop. The dotted lines are shortcuts when either more data is needed to orient on, the action is clear, or a decision is made to have another look and observe further.

The OODA loop gives us a mechanism to design systems by classifying the type of interaction and can relate to the enabling technology.

With respect to increased complexity, it allows us to focus on the now. The activities and interactions themselves are to be classified as observation, orientation, decision, or acting activities or interactions. To make sense, they always will have to form an OODA loop.

Learning together to use this way of looking at activities and interactions can increase our common understanding of complexity. In *Chapter 7, Creating New Platforms with OODA*, we will discuss in more detail how to use the model, but we will discuss the model here in terms of its relation to healthcare.

The basic idea is that observation means measuring the temperature, for example. The orientation is making diagnostics based on the measurement. If a fever is diagnosed, a decision could be made to prescribe paracetamol. The loop is closed by taking, after a while, a new temperature measurement to see if the fever has gone.

As mentioned, the model has some shortcuts. One is this: if the orientation is that the temperature is in range, further observations are done by measuring the temperature at regular intervals until a decision has to be made. This is the **observation loop**.

Another shortcut is that after orientation, we want to know if there are other symptoms to observe to get better diagnostics—for example, does the patient experience pain? This is the **diagnostics loop**.

The third shortcut is that there might be something else going on that requires a different look at the patient altogether. Maybe a different discipline is needed for a different type of treatment. This we call the **treatment loop**.

If a different discipline is needed, another team has to be involved, triggering its own OODA loop.

The following diagram shows a more elaborate OODA-loop model:

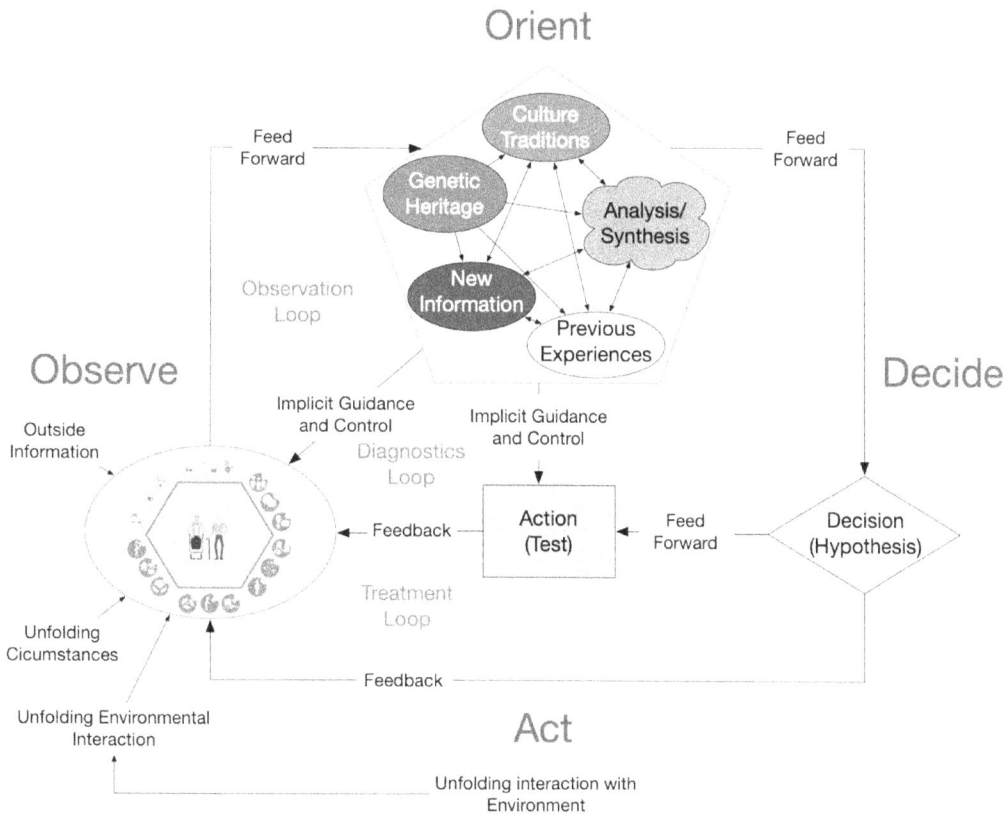

Figure 4.5 – The OODA model for sustainable healthcare

The power of the model lies in the fact that it incorporates human measures such as generic heritage consisting of the guardrails and guidelines set in medicine, cultural tradition within healthcare, and previous experiences of care workers. But the main point of OODA is that all decisions are based on observations. In the preceding diagram, we see observations coming from unfolding circumstances and interactions. Observations lead to information that is processed in the orient phase. In other words: observations do not immediately lead to decisions and actions. Observations are filtered through human factors: experience, culture, and the generic heritage of medicine. The enriched information will eventually lead to decision-making and action.

Let's elaborate this into a use case for care—a case for our TEC team. We start with the patient and observations related to the patient. The care provider will observe the health condition but will also collect data about the circumstances. That is likely raw data such as blood pressure, heart rate, body temperature, skin conditions, abnormalities in movements and cognitive capabilities, plus environmental factors ranging from weather and social activities to interactions with the caregivers in the network. A lot of this data can be collected through technical means, using medical monitoring equipment and all types of health, wellness, and activity apps. But also, the findings of other teams are observed, including their explicit decisions in the treatment loop. This data is now processed through analysis and synthesis in the orient phase and combined with knowledge, experience, and heritage to form information on the patient or patient groups on which decisions can be made.

The essence of OODA is to *get inside the OODA loop* of the health disorder of the patient. Within the observation loop, we have unfolding circumstances and interactions such as medication; hence, the care provider needs to be in control of the situation. This can be further observed, such as vital signs monitoring on the unfolding situation of health condition and circumstances, or—if needed—direct action such as changing the prescription to intervene in the situation. This implicit guidance and control take care of both normal conditions not needing extra attention and emergency situations requiring explicit action. The data gives a clear picture of what to do. Think also of the response when a fall is detected, and an alarm is forwarded.

However, if the data does not provide clear information on the situation for decisions on what to do next, we enter the diagnostics loop. At first, decisions will probably be taken on the first observations and medical history—the initial available data. Analysis and synthesis give several options to make a decision on which diagnostics are required. Think of the *Nearklinikken* **E-health Care Model (ECM)** stepped care model to decide which step to take. Prior to taking action to step up the care by a level, we can test the hypothesis by making extra diagnostics.

Are that decision and subsequent test leading to new insights? For the treatment loop, in the orient phase, the care provider needs to weigh up the outcomes—is the reaction as expected, or is it leading to new unfolding events? This can again lead to clarity for implicit control or needing another decision for a different treatment. At all phases in the loop, information must be readily available to take the right next step.

The unfolding interaction on the health journey can be precisely defined with the OODA model and used to enrich the stories. Learning about the OODA model to structure the stories is therefore recommended for specialized users such as e-nurses and developers.

It is clear by now that in the case of advanced healthcare, quick and precise data acquisition and information processing—such as diagnostics and decision support—must be designed carefully to avoid attention overload or delayed decision-making. This is increasingly the case for networked care.

Operating with OODA also means that TEC teams have to be enabled to work as autonomously as possible to be speedy with decision-making and subsequent actions based on the decisions. Teams need to be able to respond quick to unfolding circumstances: that's the essence of OODA.

The TEC teams need full support on how observations can be made and new information gathered, which protocols and procedures (genetic heritage) to follow, and which systems to use for analysis and synthesis to facilitate decision-making, to name a few. The next question is: how to organize the support for these teams? That's the third tread of TiSH. We will discuss that in the final section of this chapter.

Defining a new way of organizing healthcare

We started this chapter with systems creating a lot of various data streams, causing the risk of information overload for care providers. Next, we explored possibilities to overcome this issue by developing new systems with the use of *storytellers* and creating autonomous working TEC teams that work OODA data-driven, based on the right data at the right time and place. New systems akin to cockpits and dashboards should enable decision-making based on specific datasets and workflows.

We have one more task to do, and that is to organize these data-driven autonomous TEC teams. This can be done in traditional organizations such as a nursing home or a hospital, or with a group of practitioners. However, we saw that cooperation and collaboration between teams of what are traditionally different and siloed organizations are increasingly required to create more value. **Demolish the silos** is a remark you'll often hear when developing networked care ecosystems. Maybe it's time to look for a truly disruptive solution. Here, we need the community builders of the transformation taskforce and look at the concepts they bring in.

A solution to that challenge could be **micro-enterprises (MEs)**. At least, we invite you to think about it. In this section, we will therefore study these MEs, which allow entrepreneurship to focus 100% on the patient. We will look at the **Entrepreneurial Ecosystem Enabling Organization (3EO)** concept to organize the TEC and its supporting teams.

3EO was inspired by the **Rendanheyi** model that was first implemented by the Chinese company *Haier,* a world-leading manufacturer of domestic appliances. The **chief executive officer (CEO)** of Haier, Zhang Ruimin, is convinced that organizations constantly need to adapt to changing realities. The only way to do so is by creating network organizations that can swiftly adapt to changing conditions.

Rendanheyi literally means *employer-user-combination*, and that is exactly what the concept implies—in Rendanheyi, an employer doesn't *listen* to the one that sits higher in the hierarchy of the organization, but to the user. The user is at the center of every single decision. By doing so, organizations that work according to the Rendanheyi principles create an experience economy. It's all about the UX.

Translated to healthcare, it's all about the patient's health experience. Care organizations that adopt Rendanheyi would be better equipped to listen directly to the patients and provide care to the exact needs of the patient. The TEC teams are modeled according to the Rendanheyi principles of 3EO. They interact directly with the patients and can take joint decisions with the patients—data-driven and, as such, enabled through technology.

What Haier did with this approach was restructure its organization to become more customer-oriented. With MEs, it unbundled the organization and rebundled it into a rigorous customer-focused community.

This sounds like a good approach to focus on the health experience and a (re)constructive way to **demolish silos**.

Implementing MEs as a disruptive model in healthcare

How can we apply 3EO to organize the health experience? In *Chapter 9, Working with Complex (System of) Systems*, we will go into detail on this. For now, we will touch upon the basic principles.

It starts with the care network, as defined in the HeXagon-model that we presented in the previous chapters. This care network is the ultimate customer- (patient-) focused ME delivering the outlook on participation as value. All team members are truly focused on the care needs of the patient to achieve the optimum value.

This **HeXME** as the user ME gets revenues from insurance, the patient itself, and—as a possibility— the patient's employer and or municipality. With this revenue, formal and informal care is acquired from other MEs. This can be from local practices such as a physiotherapist's team or a **computerized tomography (CT)**-scan team residing in a hospital.

The HeXME also gets services from so-called node MEs via **shared services platforms (SSPs)** enabling support. Think of reimbursement, planning, managed IT services, getting trained on new medical methods, or career planning—typical staff operations in traditional organizations.

The value board is the **industry platform (IP)** that can decide whether user and node MEs are fitting in the ecosystem by adding the right value. The value board makes decisions based on architecture principles such as OODA-type of operations and common shared platforms design within the constraints of guardrails' value, safety, costs, and privacy.

The HeXagon elements can be found as different MEs scattered around the ecosystem and can be easily bundled and configured as required for each patient. However, to do that properly, the organizations of traditional care providers must be willing to unbundle their organization first. That probably will not start all at once, but it is possible to start with a few patients and grow from there. All transition scenarios and speeds are possible, as we will discover in the following chapters.

The 3EO system in healthcare is shown in the following diagram:

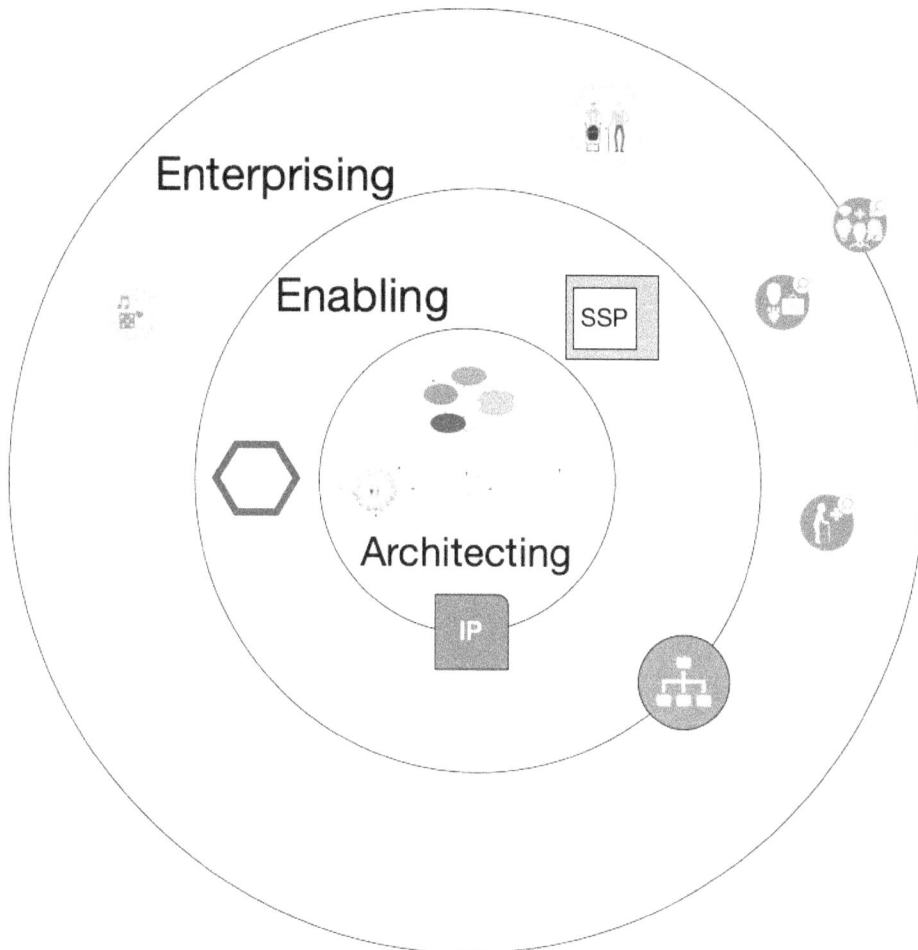

Figure 4.6 – Boundaryless 3EO map applied to health experience

In the center, the architecting takes place to ensure the genetic heritage with interoperable and integrated systems and structures throughout the ecosystem. In our case, this is symbolized by the OODA loop. Governance based on that genetic heritage is executed by the IP formed, in our case, by the value board.

The enabling-node MEs provide SSPs such as analytics services and federated regulation (blue hexagon) representing the secure exchange of medical information between MEs and staff services to nurture the culture in the ecosystem through HR, education, and coaching. The enterprising outer ring consists of specialized care teams providing care to the care network of patients.

To recap in general, 3EO is based on a few relatively simple principles for transforming organizations, as follows:

- 3EO is based on the concept of MEs as a set of loosely coupled, independent units that work autonomously, cutting down on bureaucracy and organizational debt.

- 3EO promotes a culture of independence and entrepreneurship: teams are empowered to take decisions and are responsible for those decisions. Teams can even decide to create new teams and new enterprises to fuel innovation.

- MEs are independent, but they are part of an ecosystem. Choices and strategies are derived from that ecosystem. This is likely the most important principle. In the vision of 3EO, the user shapes the ecosystem and is ultimately in charge of decisions. In healthcare, this is indeed a revolutionary model. It would mean that patients are in charge and not the care organizations.

In short, MEs have the right to make decisions and hire staff and are empowered to drive innovation. 3EO defines two types of MEs: **user MEs** and **node MEs**. User MEs directly address the needs of users—in our case, patients. Node MEs enable user MEs with more centralized functions such as **research and development** (**R&D**), logistics, and supply management. User and node MEs as a community work closely together to provide the best service that directly matches the needs of the users. User MEs also gather continuous feedback, looping back into the node MEs to constantly improve products and services.

In *Chapter 9, Working with Complex (System of) Systems*, we will study 3EO in more detail and learn more about MEs. In *Chapter 12, Executing the Transformation*, we will show how to put it all together and discuss the field experiences with autonomous teams.

Human factors in the TiSH staircase

What we have learned are the first steps in embracing complexity by introducing models to describe it. The activity triangle, interactions, workflow, OODA loop, and (re)bundling of teams can be used not only to count the number of possible interactions but also to classify them, and put them into the context of relations with guardrails, guidelines, and the value of healthcare provisioning. These are important steps to be able to get insights and use these in the transformation of healthcare.

We have studied the need for transformation in healthcare in *Chapter 1, Understanding (the Need for) Transformation*, explored new technologies in *Chapter 2, Exploring Relevant Technologies for Healthcare*, and discussed the changing roles of different stakeholders in *Chapter 3, Unfolding the Complexity of Transformation*, in that transformation—the patient being the most important stakeholder. Together with the insights based on the description of complexity, these form a basis of the requirements for transformation. It is all part of the TiSH staircase, as shown in the next diagram, which serves as a visual recap:

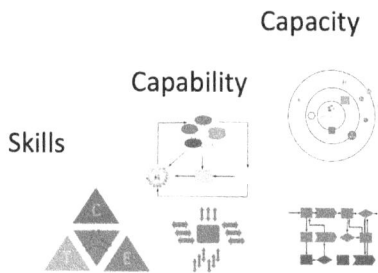

Capacity

Capability

Skills

Figure 4.7 – TiSH first three treads

The first tier shows that the Activity Theory helps in getting skilled people to interact with digital systems used in the workflows of capable teams. The second tier shows how the OODA creates capable TEC teams and takes informed decisions. The third tier is about how 3EO creates the flexibility to manage and organize the unsiloed capacity for the networked care upstairs. Together, they form building blocks to ensure the human measure in the transformation by telling compelling stories. The next chapter will complement the other building blocks of TiSH to understand how to create sustainable healthcare.

Summary

For the human factor, we learned that the Activity Theory gives us a clear point of view from people's perspectives of digital transformation. Caregivers in healthcare face a growing risk of information overload. We must create systems that allow professionals to swiftly come to the right decisions, taken jointly with and for the patient. We studied a new way of SE, focusing on UX and limiting the number of interactions between humans and systems. HSI is an architecting and engineering methodology to achieve this.

Next, these systems must be continuously improved. The same applies to processes and workflows. In this chapter, we further introduced DevOps4Care. We addressed the role of real-life storytellers to realize a process where feedback is continuously looped back into the requirements for systems, workflows, and processes, with the goal of improving the patient's life. We've studied OODA, to organize data-driven care teams. OODA teaches us how to value observations and take decisions while circumstances, such as the patient's condition, change. We learned that the right data at the right time, presented in a coherent way to the caregiver, is crucial.

Now, we need to organize teams around these data-driven concepts and make sure that these teams are mandated to make decisions. We introduced Rendanheyi and the 3EO concepts, working with MEs that form autonomously working, technology-enabled teams with an extreme focus on the patient—however, integrated into a network with other stakeholders in healthcare.

With this fourth chapter, we have learned to describe the complexity and introduced the components to eventually start working with TiSH. This will be the main subject of the next chapter—using these components as a toolkit for designing the transformation and the platform.

Further reading

If you would like to read more on the topics covered in this chapter, please refer to the following resources:

- *A Discourse on Winning and Losing, by Col John R. Boyd, USAF, Retired, Edited and Compiled by Dr. Grant T. Hammond, Air University Press, page 383 (Appendix, The OODA Loop* shows the original OODA loop)

- *Website visualizing ISO 13940, Contsys.org,* by Nicholas Oughtibridge and Trish Williams: `https://www.contsys.org/package/7+Concepts+related+to+activities`

- Blog on 3EO: `https://www.boundaryless.io/blog/an-entrepreneurial-ecosystem-enabling-organization/`

- *The Experience Economy* by B. Joseph Pine, *Harvard Business Review, 1999*

- *RenDanHeYi: the Organizational Model Defining the Future of Work?*: `https://corporate-rebels.com/rendanheyi-forum/`

5

Leveraging TiSH as Toolkit for Common Understanding

We experienced that MoM TiSH was very helpful. What more has she got in store for us?

The theme for this chapter is how to apply **Transformation in Sustainable Healthcare (TiSH)** itself. It's the core toolkit for our transformation task force to embrace complexity tread by tread. In this chapter, we will start building the TiSH toolkit for common understanding, bringing people, technology, and organizations together in a framework of comprehensible models. Eventually, this body of knowledge on models will evolve into the use of DevOps4Care, which is a specific implementation of DevOps for healthcare.

In the previous chapters, we learned that we can describe the complexity of transforming the first treads on the TiSH staircase. However, we not only want to be able to describe the complexity, but we also want to embrace it and guide the transformation itself. That is what the remaining steps on the staircase are about.

We will describe how to learn using TiSH and its underlying models and methods. TiSH and DevOps4Care will be used in the following chapters, showing you how to plan the transformation, model the digital architecture, business, and medicine for use in design, and implement innovations in healthcare and which disciplines to involve.

In this chapter, we're going to cover the following main topics:

- Starting the modeling for human-centric transformation
- Transforming for people, teams, and organizations
- Defining the transformation strategy
- Working toward automated DevOps

Starting the modeling for human-centric transformation

Transforming is about having sufficient insights into the complexity of transformation to be able to plan the next step with reasonable safety to handle the risks of not being able to predict everything. These risks are worth it because of the values to be gained, as depicted in *Figure 3.4*.

This means we need models to get insights into the complexity and models to use those insights to transform healthcare. We are going to fill the building blocks of the TiSH framework with these models and build up the embracement of complexity through common understanding tread by tread. This will be from the individual, team, and organization tiers and scales to the provisioning of care, health, lifestyle, and participation tiers and scales.

We use the **Systems of Systems Engineering (SoSE)** complexity pyramid in *Figure 3.6*, along with the DevOps4Care process steps, to get a better understanding of how all the models relate to each other. In this chapter, this will be combined in the TiSH stairway.

Let's recap what we have discussed so far. We ended with the users telling their stories comprehensibly for the developers. Now, we can put this into the perspective of the transformation.

In the first four chapters, we introduced several models. These models relate to each other with respect to the TiSH framework. Additionally, we visualized them. The visual recap is made into icons. These model icons will be used in drawings, putting the models in each other's context.

In *Chapter 1, Understanding (the Need for) Transformation*, we introduced TiSH and the objective of the transformation, participation through an optimized health experience symbolized by HeXagon, and introduced integrated care. The basic models are shown in the following diagram:

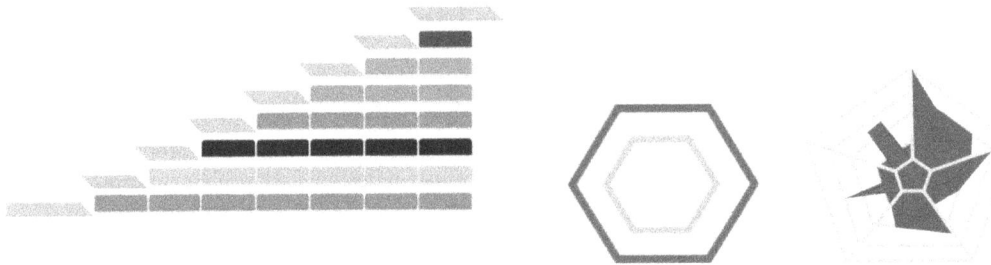

Figure 5.1 – The TiSH, directed care HeXagon, and integrated care icons

In *Chapter 2, Exploring Relevant Technologies for Healthcare*, we discussed how technology can create a data-driven network to help realize that objective. We introduced the **International Classification of Functioning, Disability, and Health (ICF)** model to represent the different types of information, discussed the stepped care model, and learned about case management. The following diagram is a visual representation of this:

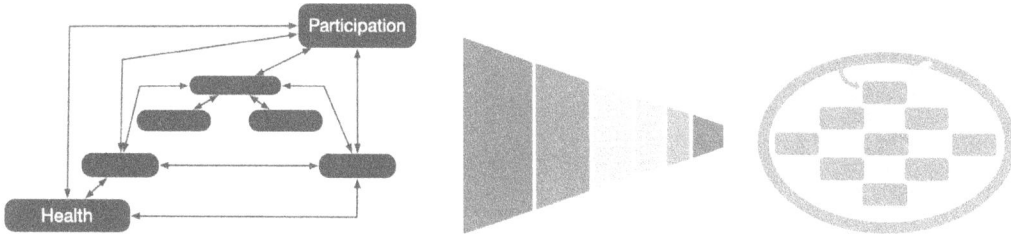

Figure 5.2 – The ICF, stepped care, and case management icons

Also, we introduced different types of technology, from standard digital input to messaging, real-world interaction with effectors, sensing in real time, the Internet of Things, AI, and autonomous robots. The icons are as follows:

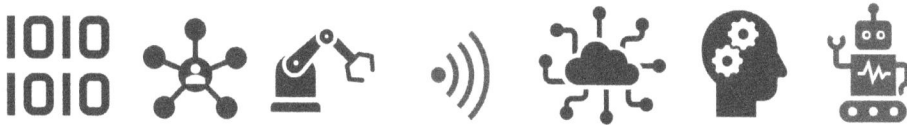

Figure 5.3 – The technology icons

Chapter 3, Unfolding the Complexity of Transformation, showed, in *Table 3.1*, the characteristics of the **4Cs** (**Communication, Coordination, Control, and Command**) and stages of networked organizations. This supports the step-by-step approach to creating value with DevOps4Care, and with the awareness that systems also increase in complexity into systems of systems. We're using the following set of icons:

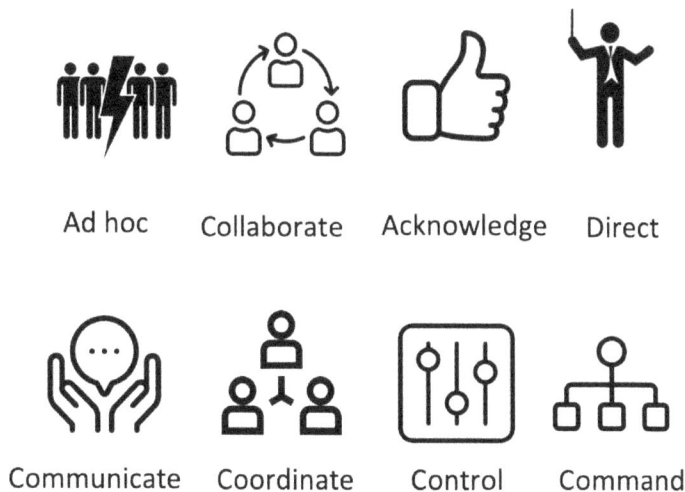

Ad hoc   Collaborate   Acknowledge   Direct

Communicate   Coordinate   Control   Command

Figure 5.4 – The 4Cs and networked organizations' icons

The visualization of value creation with DevOps4Care is shown here:

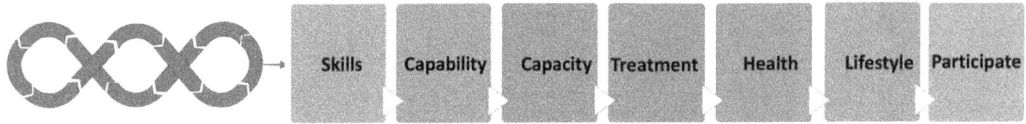

Figure 5.5 – Creating value and DevOps4Care icons

Finally, we need icons to represent the system of systems complexity and platform design. This is illustrated in the following diagram with the complexity pyramid and the a priori platform design. We need this to define TiSH as an actual complexity model that incorporates everything in the coming sections and chapters:

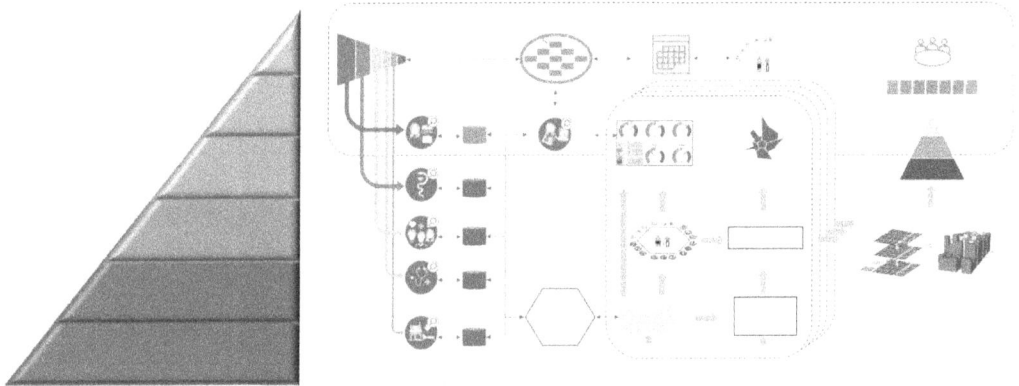

Figure 5.6 – The system of systems complexity and platform design icons

In *Chapter 4, Including the Human Factor in Transformation*, we put in the human measure at the personal level, with the activity triangle, interactions, processes and workflows, teams, and organizations, plus a way to use the **Observe, Orient, Decide, Act (OODA)** loop as the leading principal for the systems architecture. Rendanheyi is used to rebundle organizations with micro-enterprises, forming networked care in ecosystem micro-communities. The icons for the human factor are shown in the following diagram:

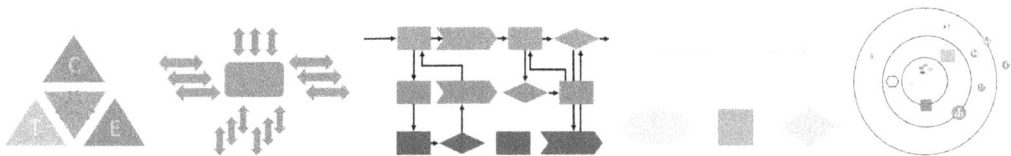

Figure 5.7 – The human factor icons

That completes all of the models so far. We have gathered a lot of the knowledge that is packed into these various models. If we continue in this way, you will probably be overloaded with even more models and knowledge. The conclusion afterward would be that the digital transformation of healthcare is indeed complex. But we promised that we can embrace this complexity to make the transformation actionable with a common understanding. That is what TiSH is all about, as we will discover in the next section.

Let's start simply with four quadrants in our reasoning framework behind TiSH, as shown in the following diagram:

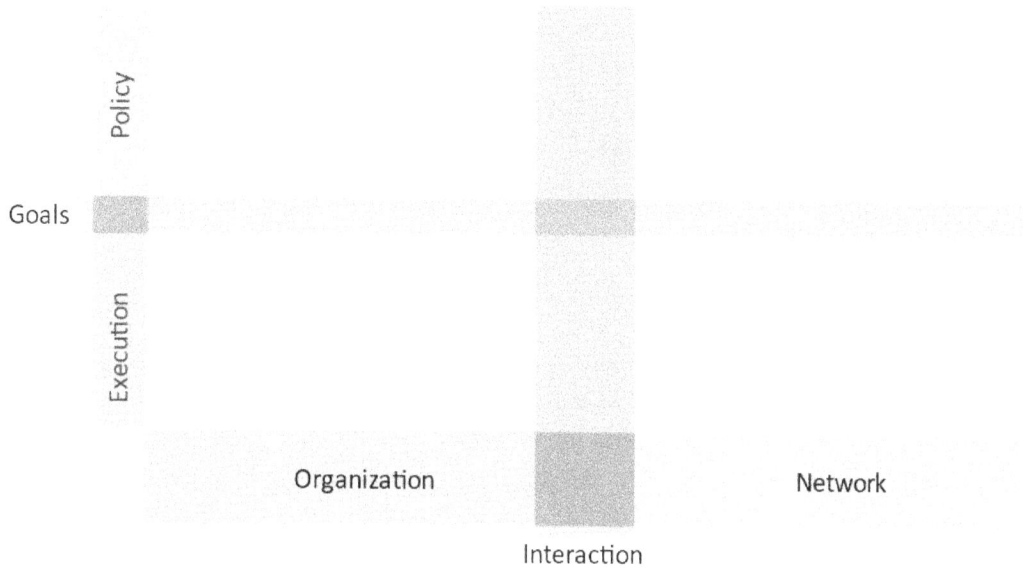

Figure 5.8 – A basic reasoning framework

The upper part is about policies, and the lower part is about execution. The left-hand side shows the internal organization, and the right-hand side shows the external network.

The overlap of **Organization** and **Network** are the interactions, and the overlap of **Policy** and **Execution** are the goals. One of the boxes in the middle is the goal for the interaction between **Organization** and **Network**.

With this basic framework, we can distinguish our reasoning between policies, execution, organization, network, and the relationship between them in terms of goals and interactions.

As pointed out, we use models for common understanding and the digital twin for **Model-Based Systems Engineering** (MBSE) at some point in the future. Let's fill the reasoning framework with the models that we presented and put them in each other's context:

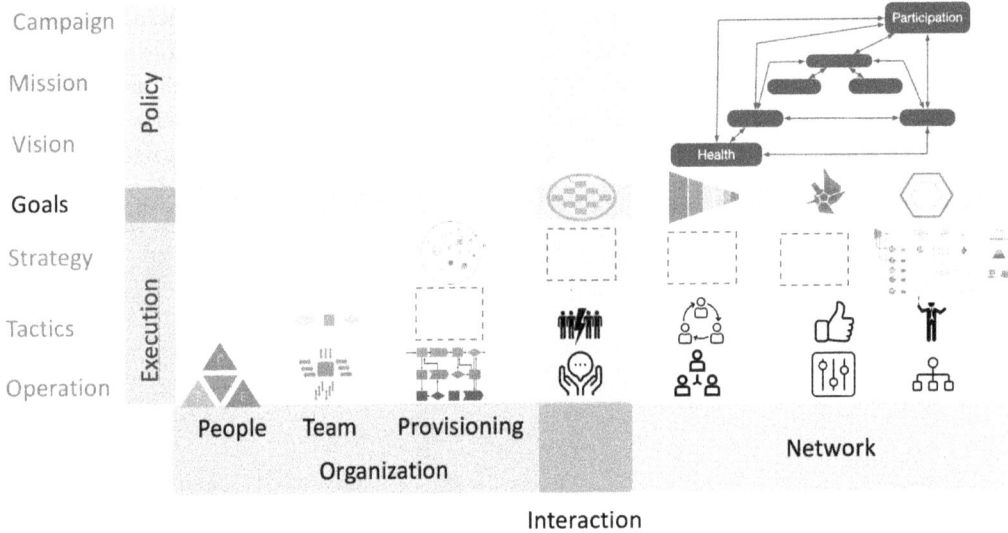

Figure 5.9 – The position of the models in the reasoning framework

The operational layer is formed by people engaging in activities, as modeled in the activity triangle, and people who interact in teams in processes and workflows for the provisioning and communicating, coordinating, controlling, or commanding of the network.

The tactical layer starts with the OODA way of working in teams, a blank for something to arrange provisioning (to be defined in *Chapter 8, Learning How Interaction Works in Technology-Enabled Care Teams* in ad hoc or virtual, collaborative, acknowledged, or directed networks.

The strategy layer begins with the (re)bundling of TEC teams for provisioning using a platform that, in the end, evolves into the solution for enabling sustainable healthcare. From the a priori solution given in *Chapter 3, Unfolding the Complexity of Transformation*, we have to define the strategy for the TEC platform for each of the goals of the four types of networked care.

If we add value creation staging, the complexity pyramid, the technology types, and DevOps4Care, then we get a better understanding of how all the models relate to each other, combined on the TiSH stairway, as shown in *Figure 5.10*.

We still have to fill in the blanks, but the models give each other the context needed to limit the complexity in each tread. For example, the first blank component is something between the TEC teams and workflows, based on OODA. Technology refers to both standard business applications and the use of effector devices such as medicine dispensers or smart locks. The value is to create capacity within a given budget. We will address that in *Chapter 7, Creating New Platforms with OODA*:

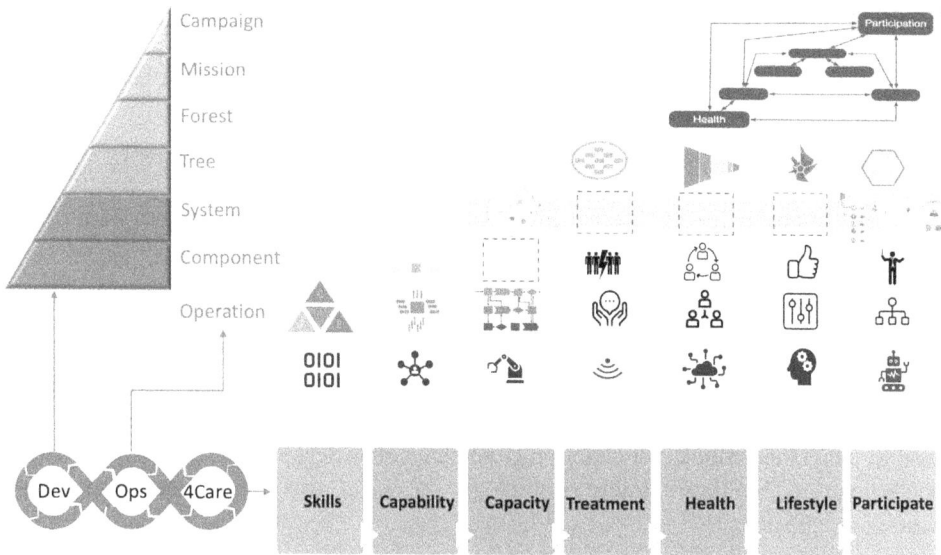

Figure 5.10 – The almost filled-in building blocks of the TiSH value staircase

The three blanks on the systems level are about the platform, which will be addressed in *Chapter 8, Learning How Interaction Works in Technology-Enabled Care Teams*, and *Chapter 9, Working with Complex (System of) Systems*. With this, we mention a quote that is allegedly from Albert Einstein: *"Keep it simple, but not simpler than that."*

In the next section, we will explore what sustainable healthcare is, what our top block campaign could look like, and what steps our transformation task force must take to achieve the goals based on our models.

Defining the campaign for transformation

A campaign needs consensus: what is the ultimate goal of transformation? Transformation is about change. But what does "change" mean? Well, it refers to something that doesn't stay the way it was, but transformation also implies that something is changing into something profoundly or even disruptively different, something that has been thought through very well indeed. Change is a consequence of choice, that is, a choice for a future direction. In the paper *Co-Emerging Futures: A model for reflecting on streams in future change*, which was published by Philips Design in 2019, this was explained in philosophical terms. A link can be found in the *Further reading* section at the end of this chapter.

One type of transformation referred to in the paper is also a sustainable (**Habitania**) scenario. Habitania aims for a good standard of living for all humans, acknowledging that the world in which humans live has limitations such as non-renewable resources. This transformation direction seeks a balance between humans and the world they live in, while also fulfilling the desire for wealth and optimal access to resources for all.

The next question, and part of setting the campaign, is *how do we get there?*

We might have an example in Society 5.0 that envisions changing healthcare in Japan to learn from.

A leading example – Society 5.0

Japanese society is facing severe threats since its population is aging rapidly, more so than in other parts of the world. This imposes massive challenges on the healthcare system. There is an urgent need to transform healthcare; first and foremost, to enable people to participate in society for as long as possible. That's the outlook that defines the campaign of Society 5.0. But secondly, the costs of traditionally organized healthcare simply get too high. The rise in costs is the second driver of the transformation of healthcare.

Japanese healthcare institutions have adopted the principles of Society 5.0 at large, shifting care to the beginning of the health continuum – prevention – using modern technology, including digitalization, and embracing biotechnology. It involves a shift from curative care to prevention, standardized care to personalized care, and provider-led healthcare to active patient involvement. The results are improved longevity with longer periods of good health and, thus, improved quality of life.

The Japanese Business Federation, Keidanren, developed an action plan for reforming healthcare in Society 5.0. This plan certainly holds some revolutionary elements, such as *unraveling mechanisms of the human body* using biotech.

The plan further comprises the mass collection, linkage, and use of life-course data:

- **Collect**: This includes genomic tests and extensive health exam checklists but also the utilization of wearable devices. The digitalization and standardization of medical and care data are key in Society 5.0.

- **Link**: Data belongs to the patient, who has control over that data through medical blockchains in **Personal Data Stores** (**PDS**) and further in the ID-controlled development of **Electronic Health Records** (**EHR**) and **Personal Health Records** (**PHR**).

- **Use**: This includes a national database forming a healthcare data platform. This platform has open access, yet is compliant with guardrails provided through new healthcare platform laws. Under these conditions and guardrails, the database can also be used by private sector firms.

The plan leads to two major developments:

- **Next-generation medicine**: This includes personalized, regenerative medicines, digital therapy, and other new forms of care.

- **Integrated healthcare services**: Personal health programs are developed providing pre-symptomatic care and prevention plans. These programs are coordinated by private firms, local governments, and hospitals. Hospitals are also involved to guide and assist in remote patient monitoring.

The closing remark in the plan of Keidanren is that *"Society 5.0 is a human-centered society. Healthcare is one domain that could benefit most through utilization of cutting-edge technologies."* This is exactly what we are trying to achieve in TiSH, using DevOps4Care.

Now we need to figure out how we can start the execution and plan the transformation. First, we need to understand that our plan doesn't stand on its own. The transformation of healthcare means the transformation of an ecosystem and the building of collaborating organizations. We will explore that in the next section. In the *Working toward automated DevOps4Care* section of this chapter, we will put it all together, connecting people, processes, and technology.

Transforming for people, teams, and organizations

It is important to understand the stories of the care workers, but also understand under which circumstances these stories have been told. The people, the teams they work in, and the organizations experience transformations that influence their stories. So, be sure to involve the management of change specialists within the task force.

We are going to explore the methods these specialists use, which can be applied to the treads of individual skills, capable teams, and organizational capacity in TiSH.

Our approach is not only about systems architecture, but also a community that enables people, teams – our **Technology Enabled Care** (**TEC**) teams – and their organizations to grow, wherein professionals learn and come to joint decision-making in a healthcare ecosystem and community:

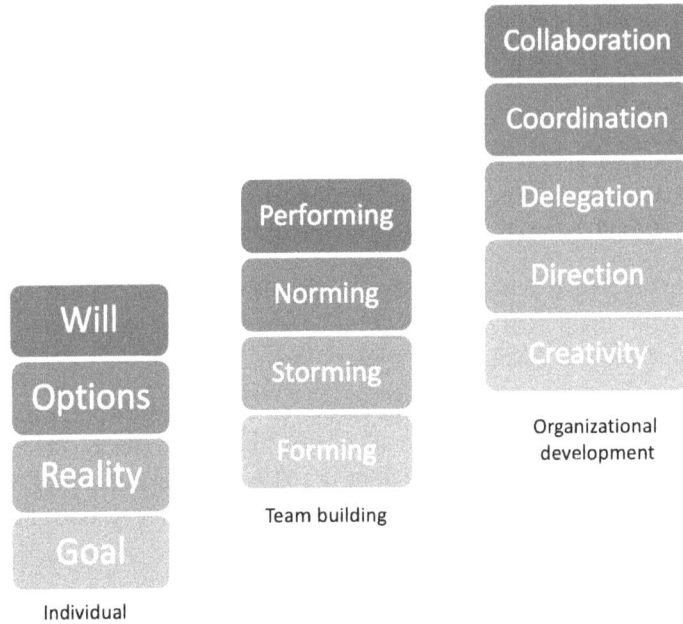

Figure 5.11 – The GROW individual model, Tuckman's team building
model, and Greiner's organizational development model

So, how do we get there? There are several methods that community builders can use for this: **GROW**, the personal growth model; Tuckman's Model of Team Dynamics; and Greiner's Organizational Growth Model. On a personal level, in the operational tier of TiSH, we can use the basic **GROW** model (**Goals, Reality, Options, Will**):

- **Goals**: What are our goals, and what do we want to achieve?

- **Reality**: What happens, and why does it happen?

- **Options**: What is the best course of action?

- **Will**: Are we provisioning the solution and executing the action (and gathering feedback to check whether we are achieving our goals)?

Our TEC teams in the tactical tier will go through the following Tuckman phases of development:

- Forming the team and getting to know each other

- Storming to establish the required relations

- Norming the purpose and goals

- Performing (the desired state)

- Adjourning when things have to be abandoned or changed

The model that Larry Greiner developed identifies five stages for growing the organization and forming a good reference for the organizational context in the strategy tier.

Greiner sees growth through the following:

- **Creativity**: This means small, informal teams that work in an agile way to create products or services.

- **Direction**: Managers are hired to give direction to the teams. Decisions are taken by managers and no longer by the teams themselves. Formal parts of an organization are formed, such as a sales or human resources department.

- **Delegation**: The leadership starts delegating tasks back to the teams and starts hiring professionals with the right skills to empower the teams. Also, responsibility is shifted back to the teams.

- **Coordination**: Teams work together to get to best results and the best outcome. Workflows and processes are matured and embedded in the culture.

- **Collaboration**: All teams work together in a trusted manner, and successes are shared amongst every member of every team. Team members are encouraged to bring in new ideas for products and services or improvements for leaner processes and workflows. All teams recognize their contribution to the success of the entire organization.

We will address these methods further in the coming chapters, such as in development cycles in *Chapter 6, Applying the Panarchy Principle*, and community building in *Chapter 11, Planning, Designing, and Architecting the Transformation*.

Defining the transformation strategy

With the changes in individuals, teams, and organizations covered, we also need specialists in the strategy of networked care. The strategy for sustainable healthcare with digital means implies that we need a TEC platform consisting of technology and the teams and communities using this technology. We need a TEC platform with modern architectures that is flexible and agile, suitable for the DevOps way of working, and that consists of reusable components from earlier treads. In technical architecture, we would refer to this as microservices – loosely coupled components that communicate with other services through interfaces. Microservices do not stand on themselves. They are all part of an ecosystem. An ecosystem exists through collaboration. So, a mature architecture is an architecture that enables collaboration in the communities. This is also true for the TEC platform.

This is only realized in a situation where user and stakeholder stories are centerstage for the DevOps4Care processes, as described in *Chapter 4, Including the Human Factor in Transformation*. Starting with the a priori solution, we need a path from the current loosely coupled digital systems of the individual care providers to the fully capable TEC platform for directed care.

Additionally, an important part of the strategy has to cope with the limited recourses of both medical and IT staff. The transformation has to facilitate autonomous self-learning systems as much as possible. The automation of DevOps4Care is a viable solution for this. Also, the transformation is about building this part of the solution. In order to do so, a model of development and operations itself is required. We will start with modeling development in this chapter. Operations will follow in *Chapter 9, Working with Complex (System of) Systems*.

So far, we have defined our own strategy to start our architecture, and we have concluded that the architecture can only mature by collaborating with and learning about organizations in the ecosystem communities of healthcare. In essence, we have laid out the strategy and the organization of the architecture of the TEC platform through collaboration, aiming for joint decision-making on all levels as the guiding process in healthcare.

Here, we need specialist knowledge from experts. Why do we ask them?

Well, for (automating) DevOps4Care and connecting to people, processes, and technology in a truly integrated architecture for every transformation, we need a structured method.

And yes, to embrace complexity, we need some sophisticated methods.

We will briefly study two possible methods used by these experts:

- **CAFCR** stands for **Customer Objectives, Application, Functional, Conceptual, and Realization**. We will use this as a decomposition of architecture.
- **Quality Function Deployment** (**QFD**) is one of the specific submethods to be applied in CAFCR to integrate or compose the architecture again.

Both methods are highly driven by user stories, which is the input that drives DevOps. Both methods work toward the definition of value, which in our case is the value for the health, lifestyle, and participation of people. We will elaborate on this in the next sections.

Working toward automated DevOps4Care

We started this chapter by looking at the reasoning framework, reflecting on TiSH and the models that we have used so far. In this section, we will learn how to use reasoning with this when working with DevOps4Care for each tread and building block on the TiSH value stairway.

In *Chapter 4, Including the Human Factor in Transformation*, we introduced the concept of user stories and the storytellers themselves as part of the 4Care part. We learned how to build a user story as a way to describe the desire of the patient and its caregivers, and what the user does or must do to achieve a certain goal.

To build the user story, we use the experience of the user, their circumstances, and the goal we want to achieve. From that user story, we derive the needs and, subsequently, set objectives and requirements to define how we must fulfill the goal and what a particular service or product should look like. In the case of the highest value tread, we consider how we should organize care to fulfill the optimal outcome and outlook for the patient. Remember our campaign: our outlook is patients, or better healthy persons, participating in society. However, experience and circumstances are equally important to each value tread.

We know that circumstances change. Therefore, we need an architecture that can adopt these changes and evolve to the next value tread. Depending on the stakeholders' perspectives, requirements might change. We constantly evaluate what happens, why events happen, what will happen, and what's the best course of action.

By doing this, we can connect the user story (human) with the DevOps process for realization using technology and work toward an accurate design of the desired solution for the chosen value. We do this with the CAFCR method, as explained next.

Reasoning is the power behind good architecting, as Gerrit Muller explains very well in his work *Architectural Reasoning Explained*. The following flowchart presents a way that tells us how to reason. We can combine this in one model that encompasses knowledge, organizational development, the human factor, and technology:

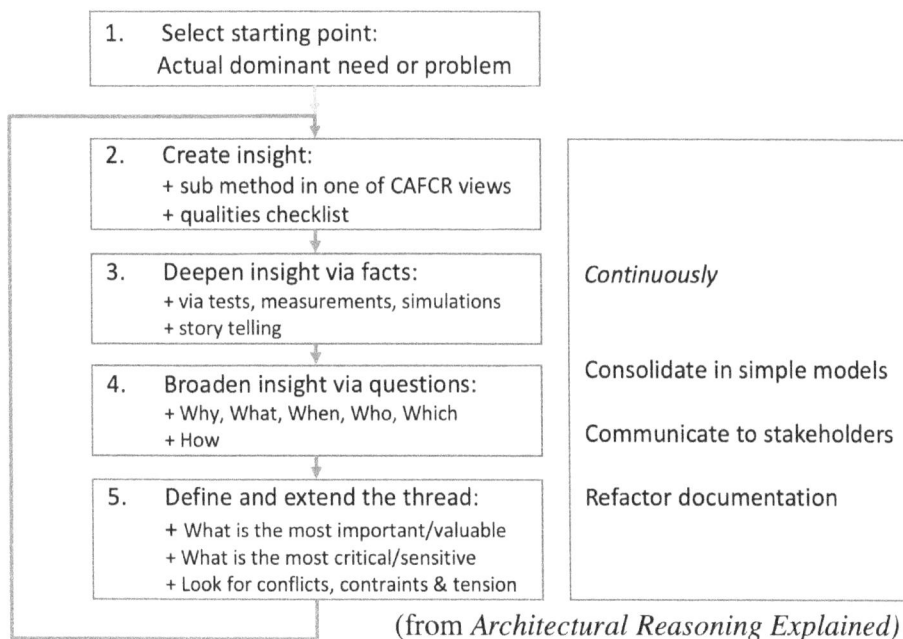

Figure 5.12 – The reasoning approach

The preceding model shows how we start from a dominant need, which, in our case, is a specific tread or building block in the transformation, to sustainable healthcare, expressed through users to create the optimum health experience in each personal HeXagon network. With this, we gain knowledge and create insights to fulfill this dominant need. These insights are broadened by asking questions such as what happens, and why does it happen? This leads to decision-making: what's the best course for action, what is influencing this course, and will these actions lead to the desired outcome? As the model shows, this is a process of continuous refinement.

In *Figure 5.13*, the CAFCR method is explained in more detail. With reasoning, you think about the design, then explore specific details, hold the details against the qualities from the guardrails and the guidelines on privacy, safety, cost and value, and use different submethods to specify the requirements of the component, system, or system of systems.

Note that, in the lower-left corner, you have the people's perspective, starting with the context of the HeXagon, and in the upper-right corner, you have the realized TEC platform. In between **Customer objectives** and **People** form the input of the application of the system (of systems) to be designed and to understand the circumstances. This is used to define the functional requirements of the system and the conceptual solutions to be realized in the actual technology to be used by the people:

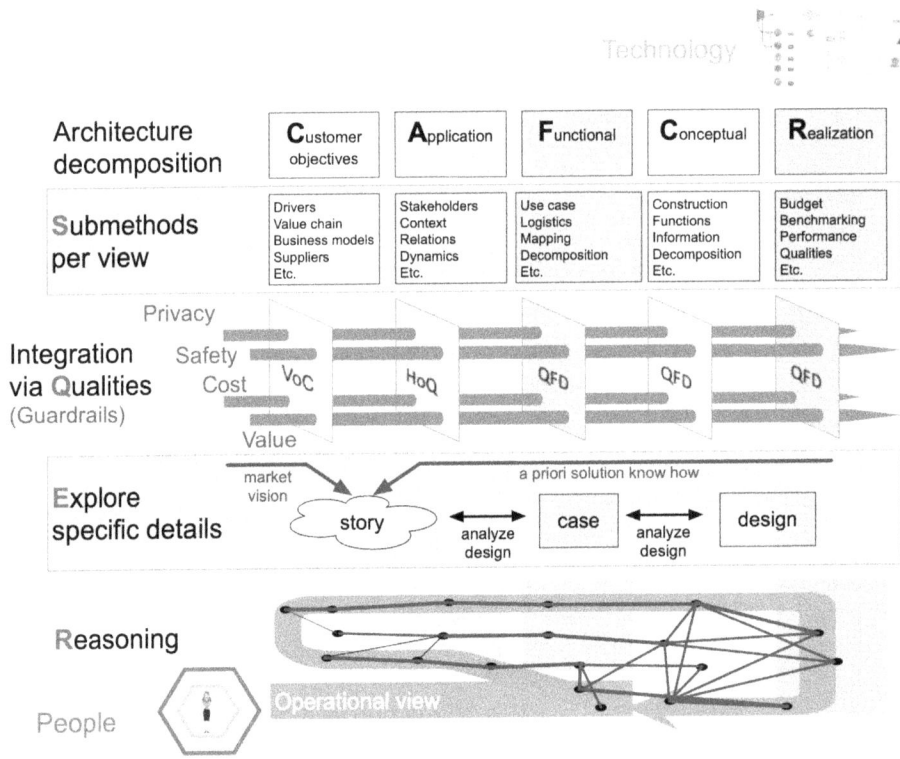

Figure 5.13 – Reasoning, exploring, qualities, and submethods using CAFCR and QFD

The power and distinction in the CAFCR method are in the four REQS layers:

- **Reasoning**: This starts with reasoning, which is probably 90% of the time spent by all involved in the development, not only architects and engineers but also operations, caregivers, and patients alike.

- **Exploring**: When it comes to sharing each other's thoughts and then stories and reflections or reactions on it are the next step to explore the needs, requirements, and possible direction of the solutions together. Design thinking workshops, patient journey sessions, prototypes, and hackathons are great ways to listen to and interact with stories, not only verbally but also by action.

- **Integrating via Qualities**: This is the rigorous process to see whether the quality standards are met via our specific application of the QFD methods, as explained next. The guardrails are mapped to architectural artifacts.

- **Submethods**: The formalization of specifications through the decomposition of artifacts is done through **Customer objectives**, **Application**, **Functional**, **Conceptual**, and **Realization** processes, logically translating the human operational view into technological realization. This is the final step that concludes the process of needs, requirements, changes, and releases.

It's fair to say that the method should be called CAFCR REQS because the four REQS layers are at the core of the model.

Reasoning is mostly done individually. Exploring is done jointly via the user stories. We have already paid some attention to both. Integrating the qualities and formalizing specifications using submethods also have to be addressed with formal models to embrace the complexity, by keeping consistent and being comprehensible, and being able to automate the DevOps4Care cycles.

The models forming the building blocks form a starting point.

Remember that, in our reasoning threads, the viewpoint of the customer objectives must be derived from health experiences. That requires a relation map. That relation map could look like the diagram in *Figure 5.14*. Here, the QFD map comes in and represents the integrated architecture, connecting people with processes and technology in which the CAFCR elements can be recognized:

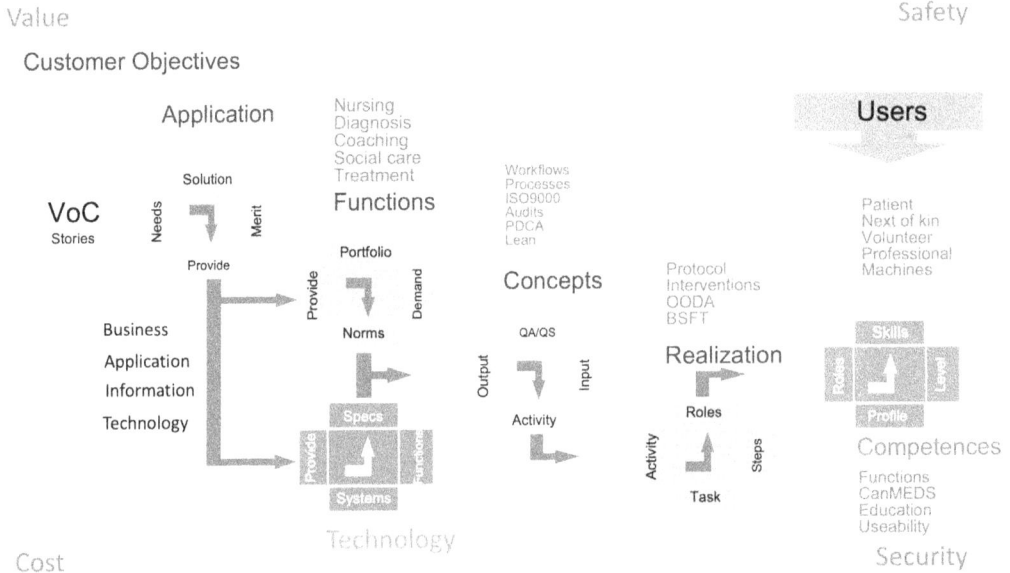

Figure 5.14 – Going from Customer Objectives to Realization and back to Users

Clearly, we start with the users, who are the patients, but also the next of kin, professional caregivers, and volunteers helping to provide care. The user is everyone and everything that can be seen as an entity or actor that plays a role in providing (think of devices, too) or receiving care.

Users have competencies: they have a profile and a specific role, and through education and experience, have gained the skills to perform a function. One way to define a profile is through the **Canadian Medical Education Directions for Specialists (CanMEDS)** framework that identifies the abilities that practitioners require or **Skills Framework for the Information Age (SFIA)** 8 for IT competencies.

From the different user perspectives, we derive user stories to identify customer objectives. Remember that we must deal with various dimensions: a society where users live, organizations that they are part of, and their skill levels of using technology, just to name a few examples. All of this matters in terms of defining the user story and, eventually, setting objectives. What type of care is required? What type of care must be provided? This translates into the **Voice of the Customer (VoC)**, which we will discuss, in more detail, in the next section.

From the VoC, we can define the solutions using the other steps of CAFCR. Customer objectives are translated via a **House of Quality (HoQ)** into requirements following the **BAIT** principles: **Business, Application, Information, Technology**. A business requirement answers the following question: what problem are we solving? To understand the problem and define the solution, we need information. The interface to that information – data – is the application.

To support users to get information using an application, we need technology: a comprehensive tool to view and analyze data that enables the execution of functions. Functions are assembled in a portfolio providing solutions for prevention, diagnostics, treatments, and different forms of care.

> **Note**
>
> To get a better understanding, please read the classic article, *House of Quality*, by John R. Hauser and Don Clausing, which was published in May 1988. It can be found on HBR at `https://hbr.org/1988/05/the-house-of-quality`.

Now we need people to work with that portfolio, providing solutions that match the objectives and requirements of the customer. For that, we use the models in *Figure 5.14*.

Besides that, patient safety and security are a priority when it comes to providing care, next to costs and value. Hence, we need guardrails to make sure that care is provided safely by people that have the right knowledge and skills to execute the solutions at affordable costs with respect to the value experienced. These professionals along with the patients will give feedback on the solutions. This feedback is looped back into the VoC, completing the life cycle of DevOps4Care.

By the way, what we just did is reasoning through QFD threads. We started reasoning from the customer, translated that into objectives and requirements, defined a methodology to derive solutions, and made sure that we created a safe, secure environment to execute those solutions. In the next section, we will explain how to use QFD and HoQ more specifically.

Here, we remark that the experts included in the transformation task force must be given time to exercise these methods in the task force to make the task force more capable.

Using the VoC in DevOps

In the previous section, we introduced the VoC to define customer objectives and as a methodology to start creating user stories. VoC is part of a broader method called QFD. In this section, we will explore what QFD is and how it can help us in transforming healthcare.

Once we have defined the user story, we must integrate it with the constraints of the stakeholders so that we specify the exact requirements. For exploring constraints and translating to specifications, QFD is a comprehensive method. QFD is a process that helps to translate customer requirements into the detailed specifications of products, by describing the various components and planning of development, tracking the entire process to ensure that the requirements are fulfilled.

The HoQ is another attribute within QFD to ensure that the customer requirements (VoC) have a direct relationship with the activities to achieve these requirements. The HoQ is a quality matrix that monitors whether the requirements are met and how resources are planned to fulfill the requirements in Dev, Ops, and 4Care.

In QFD, it is essential how the VoC is communicated throughout an organization. The entire organization needs to be aware of the VoC to work together in creating the desired products and services that deliver value to the customer, expressed in the VoC. QFD emphasizes the demands and wishes of the customer, which need to be accomplished. It does not focus on what a provider believes a customer wants or desires.

So, how does this match with DevOps principles and user stories? Well, a user story could be a good way to make the VoC tangible and very concrete. Where, in DevOps and agile, we would get to the so-called epics and features of the product, QFD defines four stages in getting to the definition and development of a product or service. Also, user stories must come from real voices, not what an engineer thinks the user wants!

With this in mind, we will study the four stages briefly, mapping them to DevOps and agile artifacts:

- **Product definition**: This is based on the collection of the VoC. In agile working and DevOps, we would define an **epic**, which is an artifact that can be detailed in specific tasks – the user stories – based on the needs and demands of the customer.

- **Product development**: Components of the product are identified and specified. In DevOps, we would refer to **features**.

- **Process development**: In this phase, the process flow is developed, describing how the product is being assembled.

- **Quality control**: The product is tested and inspected for any failures. Only when all the tests have been successfully completed, the product is launched for production. Testing for quality is essential in DevOps. This is always a team effort. The team defines and designs the tests and decides when tests have resulted in the expected outcome. The HoQ plays an essential role in this process. So, have these activities led to the desired outcome?

We can translate that to healthcare and DevOps4Care. We start with the VoC, and using the HoQ, we monitor whether all activities lead to the desired outcome, which is health to participate in society (again). Through aligned processes, team participation, and integrated workflows we ensure collaboration. In *Chapters 7*, *8*, and *9*, we will learn how to make this specific.

Take another look at *Figure 5.14*: you will now recognize how VoC, HoQ, and QFD provide quality guardrails. Now that we have a place for our guardrails, we are ready to start the execution of the transformation. The next step is this: getting everyone on the same page in terms of shared mental models at the same time in the following chapter.

Summary

In this chapter, we worked toward using the TiSH staircase and its building blocks. We started by looking at each perspective of the different models in the transformation. Next, we used this for defining our campaign and setting goals. Our campaign is providing the outlook for patients, which is participation in society.

The strategy to enable the operations and tactics in the care networks is set by defining a TEC platform – a platform that has to be developed and operated by IT personnel and used by people involved in care.

Guided by reasoning in the reasoning framework, we next defined the steps that we must take to achieve the goals of this campaign. In this chapter, we worked with various models and methods that help us in defining these steps, forming the teams to execute the steps, and understanding what skills are needed to provide care in a new, disruptive manner. It all started with applicable models for each building block: we have to know where we are coming from and where we are going, along with what our final destination is. That defines the transformation.

We learned that needs and requirements are crucial in defining each of the transformation phases. We are aware that specialists are needed to do this. We studied the methodologies they use to gather these requirements wherein the demands of the patient are the priority. Methodologies such as CAFCR and QFD with the HoQ and the VoC are coherent ways in which to grasp the requirements.

The essence of TiSH is to get care professionals to work together in teams, where they jointly decide with the patient what the best course of action is, given the circumstances and the desired outlook of that patient. Technology can be of great aid, but we need to train professionals in working with technology to get the best results in the different stages of care. In other words, care teams, supported by technology, jointly decide with the patient what the desired value is in the outcome of care processes. Therefore, technology, people's roles, and organizations have to be designed and developed together in a community to realize the required value.

In the following chapters of this book, we will start the execution of this process using the models and methods that we put into perspective in this chapter.

Further reading

- Paper on transformation by Philips Design, 2019: `https://www.researchgate.net/publication/333972702_Co-Emerging_Futures_A_model_for_reflecting_on_streams_of_future_change`

- The action plan of the Japanese institute, Keidanren, for Society 5.0: `https://www.keidanren.or.jp/en/policy/2018/021_overview.pdf`

Part 2: Understanding and Working with Shared Mental Models

Shared mental models are about having a shared understanding among team members and their multidisciplinary stakeholders about how they should behave in different situations. How is this relevant to healthcare and specifically the transformation of healthcare? The success of a transformation is defined by a common understanding of the needs and goals for that transformation. It sets the requirements for architecture and the transformation strategy.

The following chapters will be covered under this section:

- *Chapter 6, Applying the Panarchy Principle*
- *Chapter 7, Creating New Platforms with OODA*
- *Chapter 8, Learning How Interaction Works in Technology-Enabled Care Teams*
- *Chapter 9, Working with Complex (System of) Systems*

6

Applying the Panarchy Principle

Acquiring knowledge at school is one thing, but we also have to learn what the real world is like. MoM TiSH introduces us to the dynamics of society.

So far, we have discussed the need for transformation, a platform, a transformation task force, and new skills in systems engineering and community building disciplines in this task force. We filled our toolbox to model this transformation. However, to be effective, this requires getting everyone on the same page regarding the shared mental models so that they can move from one tread to the next.

In this chapter, we will look at community building. The engineering and medicine disciplines in the task force need to understand the dynamics of community building and how to take it into account when designing new technology-enabled care platforms.

Where we pointed to INCOSE for great resources on systems engineering, we will also refer to the systems innovation network for community building. First, we will introduce the ecocycle and panarchy models and introduce supporting ecocycle submethods to define the dynamics of community building. This will provide a brief overview of awareness on the dynamics of change on all levels, though one chapter is not enough for a deep dive.

Then, we will learn how to use the principle of interdependent ecocycles to determine people's states of mind and help plan the transformation. Overcoming inhibition is important in ecocycles as it might slow down the transformation.

In this chapter, we're going to cover the following main topics:

- Transitioning from tread to tread
- Understanding ecocycles and panarchy
- Applying the panarchy principles to TiSH
- Understanding people's state of mind

Transitioning from tread to tread

This is a good moment to have another look at the TiSH staircase that we presented in the previous chapter. In that model, we presented treads and stages of transformation. What we haven't discussed in that model was *how* to get from one tread to another. This is where transformation hits: with every step that we take to the next tread, we will find that these treads are rollercoaster rides. We need to carefully plan and time our ride and be aware of the fact that it will move at different speeds as circumstances such as bends, loops, and hills will change. The TiSH staircase might appear as something in which we can plan everything, but the reality is that we can't always plan where *our feet are concerning our heads* on every step.

We take this rollercoaster metaphor to symbolize the dynamics of change. These dynamics have different grounds but people's state of mind is something that can be determined; then, these insights can be used to define the transitions taken in the transformation:

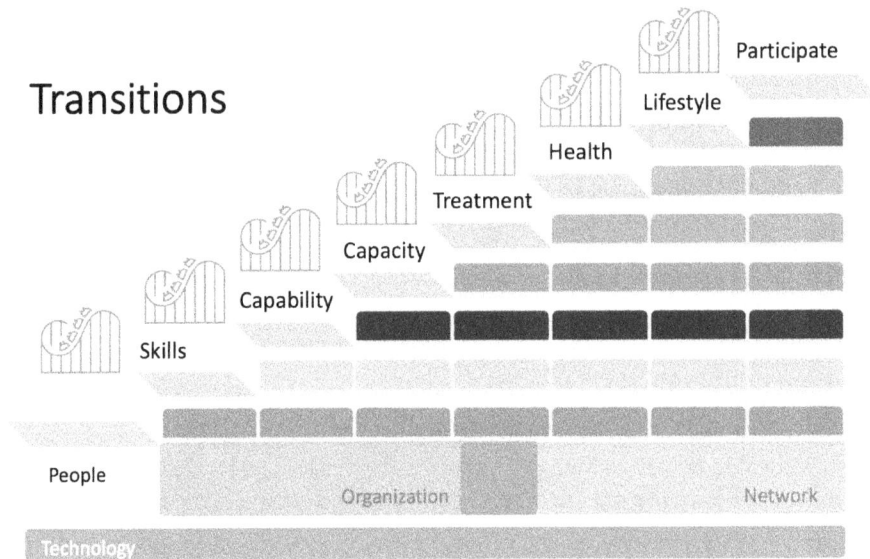

Figure 6.1 – Transition rollercoaster for each tread

Each higher tread means growing in scale with each transition. This starts with individuals and then ever bigger groups of people with new goals to achieve.

The first tread is the transition to having enough people with the right digital skills. The second is the transition to capable TEC teams, the third is the transition to enough capacity, and so on. If the transformation can be done tread by tread, then this is manageable, but what we see in the real world is that the transitions on all treads take place simultaneously at different speeds. These transitions also influence each other. If people are not skilled enough, then this will inhibit the transition on higher treads. Another example is that if the rules on health values are not clear, this will cause certain treatments not to be reimbursed. The transitions influence each other from both sides.

We need to understand the rollercoasters on each transition and how they influence each other for a successful transformation. This is where ecocycles and panarchy come in.

Understanding ecocycles and panarchy

The metaphor of the rollercoaster needs some more definition to be practical; we need to know more than that it could be a bumpy ride ahead. Therefore, we must introduce the generic ecocycle model to determine people's and the organization's state of mind:

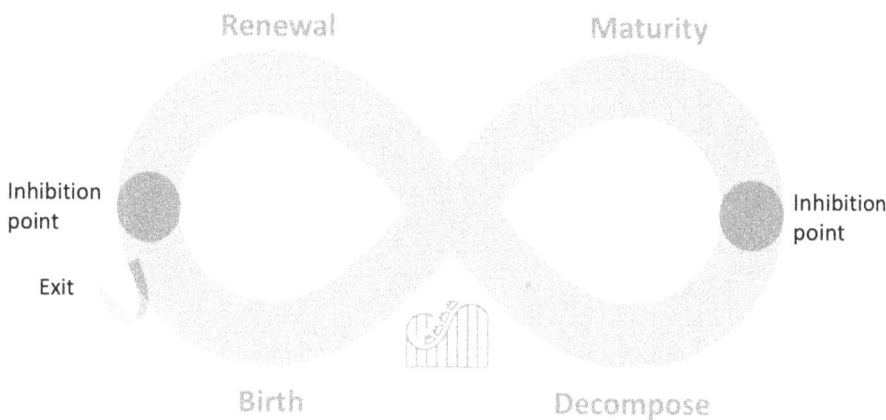

Figure 6.2 – The adaptive ecocycle

This ecocycle can be viewed as a rollercoaster, which consists of the following four states of mind:

- **Maturity**: Things are continuing as usual; there's no need for change
- **Decompose**: The old has to go; something new is needed
- **Renewal**: New ideas are explored
- **Birth**: New ideas are put into practice and grow toward the new normal

There are also two inhibition points. The inhibition point on the right denotes not letting go of the old. People feel that something has to change but do not make the step to do so. The inhibition point on the left denotes not deciding to invest in the new way. People know what to do but experience a lack of funding.

Different people tend to be in different states of mind, and not all states are fruitful enough to invest time into building new common understanding. The urgency for change must be commonly felt. It's in the **Renewal** state that common understanding has the best opportunity to change.

This ecocycle can be applied to all scales of people and all transitions, from the individual using the technology to groups of people in teams, organizations, and networked care forms:

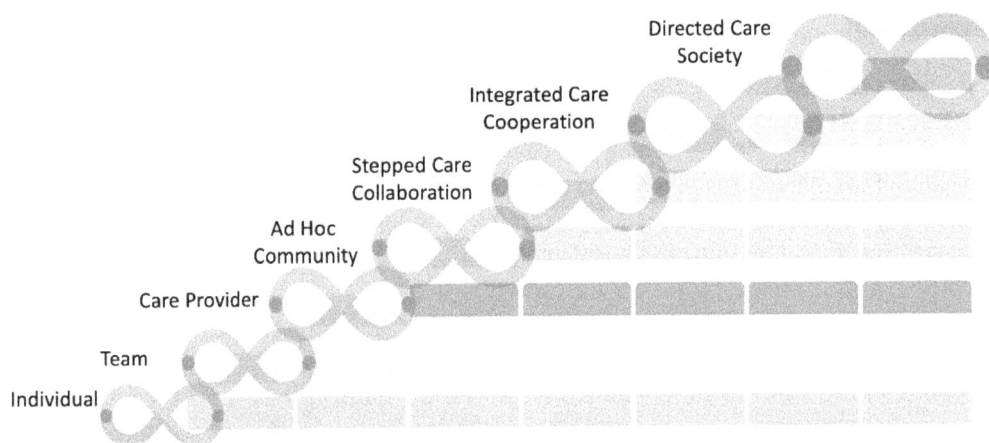

Figure 6.3 – The adaptive ecocycle on all TiSH scales

Determining where on each scale the prevailing state of mind is and where the inhibitions points are will help in planning the transformation.

This way of viewing complex systems is called a panarchy, a complex study that seeks to explain how economic growth and human development interact and depend on ecosystems and institutions. In our experience, we have applied this to healthcare too: assessing the (global) growth in healthcare and how ecosystems in healthcare interact with each other. Something key in panarchy is the adaptive ecocycle: how do individuals and groups adapt to changing circumstances across the scale from individuals and departments in healthcare institutions to networks in the societal ecosystem?

In our situation, the vast potential of technology plays a significant role in this. Some of these technological circumstances can be influenced; others can't. What is the overall impact on healthcare and how can we deal with this in the transformation? Panarchy is, as mentioned previously, complex, but in this chapter, we will try to explain how it's relevant to the transformation of healthcare and how it gives insight into the design and helps execute the transformation.

We need insights into creating an understanding of how to model the behavior of individuals, teams, organizations, and networks in different circumstances and situations. Simply put, how can we get people in organizations, teams, and team members, as well as their clients and suppliers, on the same page and get them to share a common understanding on how they achieve goals?

People will find themselves confronted with circumstances that develop faster than they can comprehend. They will discover that networked care will increasingly become more important and how technology is accelerating that. The development of technology might be faster than teams can absorb. This is exactly what the concept of panarchy and ecocycles can model and describe.

> **Tip**
>
> To learn more about panarchy as a concept, we recommend reading a paper by Paul. B. Hartzog entitled *Governance in the Network Age*. His definition of panarchy is *complexity + networks + connectivity = panarchy*. He describes panarchy as an emerging complexity of social and political structures that continuously form new networks that interact with each other and are supported or even propelled by technology. The forming and the levels of interaction take place at various speeds, causing some networks to be more advanced and others to lag. This is what we see today in healthcare at different scales: individual, local, regional, national, and even global.
>
> Other sources where you can learn more include *Panarchy: Understanding Transformations in Human and Natural Systems*, by Gunderson and Holling, and the Ecocycle Planning section of the Liberating Structures website, `https://www.liberatingstructures.com/31-ecocycle-planning/`.

To be able to understand the dynamics of the panarchy, we are building on the basic ecocycle. First, we must add some extra characteristics for each stage of the ecocycle and the roles involved:

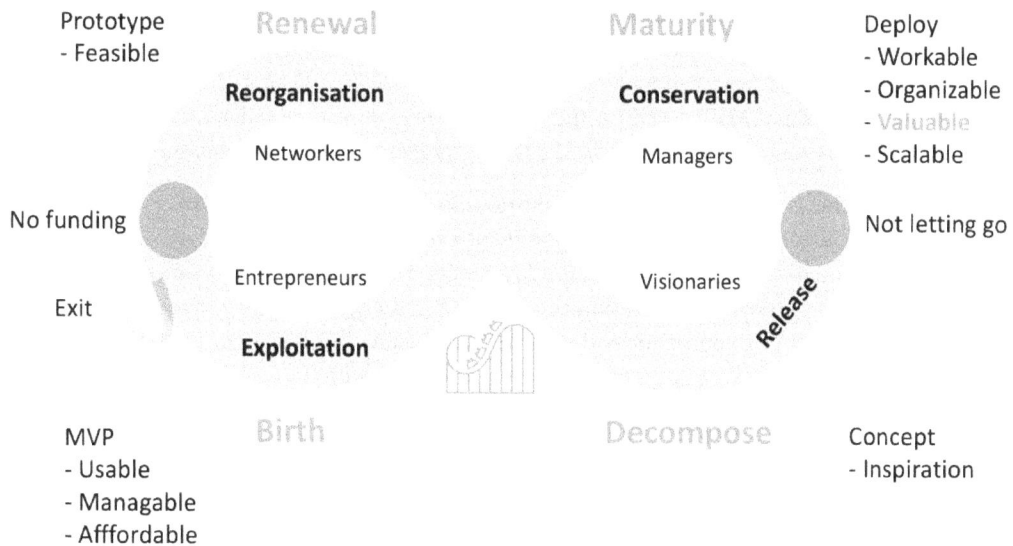

Figure 6.4 – The adaptive ecocycle – stages, roles, and criteria

The four stages in the adaptive ecocycle are as follows:

- **Exploitation**: This is the phase of birth and fast growth. Here, we can think of the introduction of new technology and/or a way of working in a society that is rapidly adopted by a population.

- **Conservation**: In this stage, we see stabilization; for example, the new technology is adopted by a larger population and, as such, maturing because they see the benefits and value.

- **Release**: The growth declines because, for example, the populations need changes that require different technologies or, due to changed circumstances such as a different attitude to privacy, populations abandon the new technology or service as a whole, seeking something new to fulfill the changed requirements.

- **Reorganization**: This is about renewal. Because of changed conditions such as demographics, the technology needs to be renewed to address the new circumstances. From this point onward, the cycle starts over again or exits.

Each stage has different people involved with different roles. Exploitation is led by entrepreneurs who start – or give birth – to new endeavors; the managers mature the endeavor and conserve its advancements. In this stage, it takes a creative visionary to become the game-changer who releases themselves from conserved thinking by decomposing the new needs into new possibilities. The networkers integrate new possibilities to renew the available solutions and enablers. These renewed possibilities inspire entrepreneurs.

Each of these roles has a different perspective and criteria they look at. The visionary is looking for inspiration and ideas, whereas the networker seeks the feasibility of the idea, preferably with a prototype or proof of concept. The entrepreneur looks at usability, manageability, and affordability, starting with a **Minimal Viable Product** (**MVP**), whereas the managers are looking to see whether the platform is workable, organizable, valuable, and scalable. The term *valuable* relates to our value stages.

Another characteristic is that the stages do not take up equal time, nor do they behave as clockwork. Think of Exploitation and Conservation as the lift hill of a rollercoaster (*Figure 6.4*). A ratchet clicks with every advancement to assure the gained improvements. The Release and Reorganization stages are more like the rest of the track, providing enough kinetic energy to complete the entire course under a variety of disrupting conditions and start the cycle again. This metaphor gives insight into two crucial points on the track: the release point on top of the hill, with the option of not letting go if it's not safe, and boarding the new ride. Who wants to buy or invest in new tickets? Both can inhibit the carts to move further.

These inhibition points are influenced by the ecocycles of the other treads. As shown in *Figure 6.5*, these connections make up the panarchy:

- From new ideas in the Release stage to the last phase of the Conservation stage one tread up, the revolution from below accelerates the transformation

- From the experience gathered in the Conservation and Renewal stages, the tread acts as a conservative force, which decelerates the transformation from above:

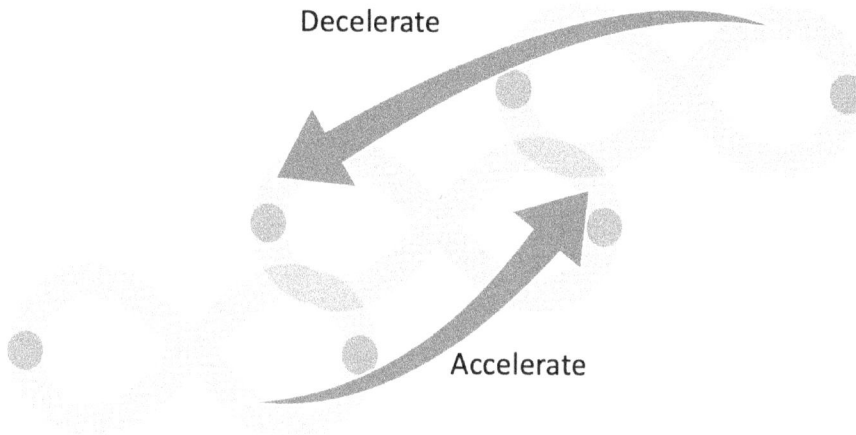

Figure 6.5 – The panarchy connections

For example, if a new technology is picked up by a visionary, this can trigger the team if they are at the end of the Conservation stage and starting to come across dilemmas. Only then will they consider this new technology and let go of the current way of working.

If the team does let go and comes up with a new way of working, it's the next inhibition point that has to be overcome before the Exploitation stage can begin. The organization's previous experience, culture, and heritage will influence the team in the Renewal stage and probably tell them that value must be created for the organization. In our case, this is the capacity to provide reimbursable health services. If the organization itself is in another stage of its ecocycle, it becomes less clear what the influence is. A natural way is when the ecocycles synchronize where they overlap in the panarchy. If the individuals already have the right skills for the new technology, it's easier to start the Exploitation stage in the team to build their capabilities. When that is matured, this can form the basis to start building enough capacity in the organization.

With these loosely coupled but further independent dynamics of each tread ecocycle, the transformation task force will not be able to plan the transformation. What it can do, however, is understand the dynamics and use those dynamics to facilitate transitions when the timing is right.

Understanding is also key to driving each ecocycle. The task force can facilitate common understanding activities with the methods presented in this book or others if they're more suited for the specific situation.

It's the task force that must identify these stages and act with common understanding activities when the time is right.

On an amusing note, it can be said that the task force has to wait for the right alignment of planets on their cycles, just like an astrologist does.

Planning the ecocycles

Technology releases can occur daily, but learning new skills takes weeks. Applying these skills to the teams takes months, (re)organization takes many quarters, and networked care can take years to a decade. However, we can accelerate the cycle times by creating a common understanding.

Here is how to achieve this:

- Determine in which ecocycle stage each tread is.
- Plan and execute common understanding sessions with the shared mental models suitable for each tread.
- Involve the treads below and above the panarchy to help the accelerators trigger the release and the decelerators avoid not getting funded, respectively. This must be aligned with the stage of the ecocycle as shown with the blue arrows in *Figure 6.5*.
- Use common understanding to agree on the transitions required and make plans accordingly.

Now that we are aware that ecocycles and panarchy help us understand people's state of mind and the growing pains of change, let's learn how this helps us further understand the complexity of transformation in healthcare. We will do that in the next section.

Applying the panarchy principles to TiSH

We will start this section with a general remark that applies to almost every transformation, but specifically to digital transformation. Typically, technology moves faster than the organizations that need to adopt the technology. Healthcare is no exception to this rule. However, transformation is a journey. It requires a plan and planning to get where you want to be as an individual, team, organization, or network, which helps you define what you need to complete the journey. That's where the TiSH staircase comes in: it describes the different *transitions* in that journey.

With every transition to a new tread, we must prioritize, balance, and consider viewpoints while focusing on the bigger picture, which is the ultimate goal that we are trying to achieve. Let's take the necessary steps.

The challenge is that DevOps development and releasing the new technology will potentially be faster than the adoption of that technology in organizations and society at large. We can see this in the TiSH staircase: every person that is confronted with new technology must go through a transition, as well as all the treads above that. If we do a release from DevOps, we must consider how this is impacting the treads in the staircase. Monitoring the stories on perceived value on all treads becomes the essential source for renewal.

From the bottom up of the TiSH staircase, we have technological revolutionary forces driving innovation; from the top down, we will be confronted by constraining forces that simply need time to understand and adapt to the innovation. The power of TiSH is having a common understanding – with shared mental models – to achieve the goals. The key is that technology accelerates the (eco)cycle time, which can lead to revolution (fast adoption) when needs are understood well.

To understand when those needs surface and can or will be told, we can use the ecocycles in the panarchy from bottom to top. This will help with the DevOps part of the platform with a needs-based release as it will know when and how to listen based on the following:

- Individuals that recognize their state of mind

- Teams in their development state

- The organization stage

- The care networks stage

Let's explore the panarchy for this purpose.

Defining the individual ecocycle

The first thing technology encounters on the TiSH staircase is the individual user and their ecocycle. Let's have a closer look at how people adopt innovations. We have chosen to use the Mezirov model for that. It describes the transformational learning phases a person goes through in adopting innovations:

1. **Disorientation**: A dilemma that challenges the current normal situation.
2. **Self-Examination**: Reflect on the current situation; is it sustainable?
3. **Critical Assessment**: Question whether previously held beliefs are future-proof.
4. **Relating**: Recognize you are not alone.
5. **Exploration**: Possibilities in the new situation, new roles, and relationships.
6. **Planning**: Plan to implement the changes.
7. **Knowledge**: Strengthen your skills and learn what you need to adapt.
8. **Experimentation**: New roles and ways of working.
9. **Self-Confidence**: Built competence and capabilities (group).
10. **Reintegrate**: The new way of data-driven working as the new normal.

We can plot these phases onto our ecocycle pattern, as shown in the following diagram:

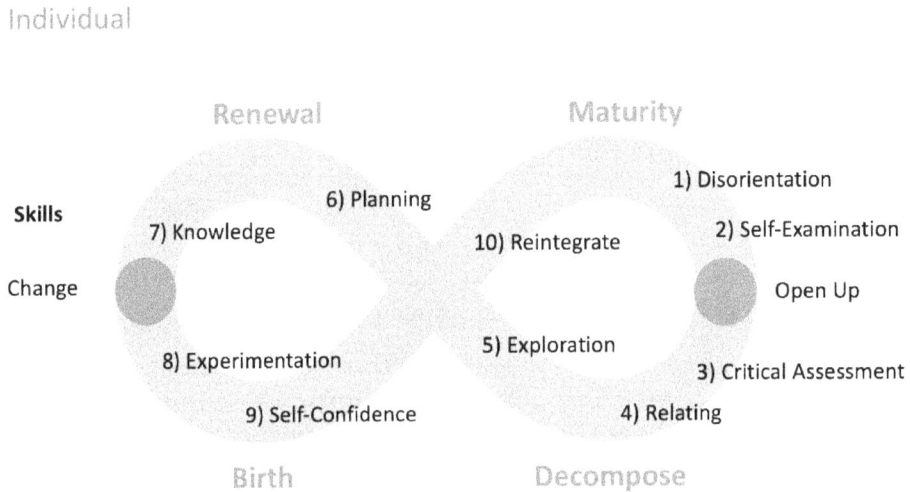

Figure 6.6 – The individual ecocycle

What is the connection between technology and this individual ecocycle? The influence between the ecocycles is complex but can be modeled in such a way that we can apply our reasoning to it.

But how do individuals get caught in a dilemma? This happens because they are team members. It's the transformation of the teams where the dilemmas originate.

Note that from the exploration learning phase, the individuals can influence the teams they are part of to accelerate the team ecocycle. On the other hand, if the team is performing well, it can inhibit how newly gained skills are applied to the experimentation phase.

Common understanding can be improved by organizing **Observe, Orient, Decide, and Act (OODA)** sessions to build a shared mental model of how technology can help organize healthcare at the activity level. To determine what topics should be addressed in such sessions, the Activity Triangle can be used as a template.

Defining the team ecocycle

If we move one level up to the teams, we can look at Tuckman's model of Team Dynamics. We discussed this model in *Chapter 5, Leveraging TiSH as Toolkit for Common Understanding*. Tuckman describes how teams go through different stages – forming, storming, norming, performing, and adjourning – to get to know each other and then jointly define how the purpose and goals can be best met as a team. The team ecocycle is shown in the following diagram:

Team

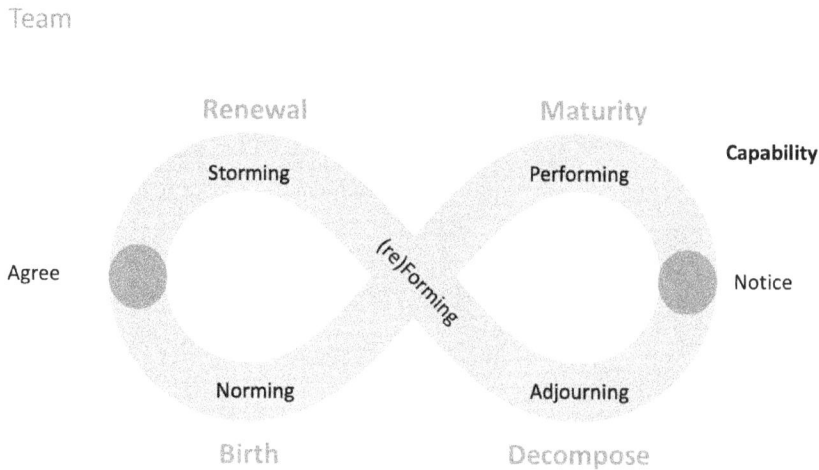

Figure 6.7 – The team ecocycle

The step from adjourning to (re)forming is the point at which the organization's influence can cause the current way of working to be released. Note that not all teams will go through this cycle at the same time. It will probably start with a more progressive team in the organization.

The organization can influence the inhibition point to let the team agree on new norms if the organization does not see how their value in increased capacity would be realized.

The task force can organize common understanding sessions on customer or health journeys to discover the value of teams working with new forms of technology at the touchpoints on that journey.

Defining the organization ecocycle

The next level is organizations. For this, we can use Rendanheyi again. We discussed the concept of Rendanheyi in *Chapter 4, Including the Human Factor in Transformation*, where we described it as an organization wherein the employer doesn't *listen* to the one that sits higher in the hierarchy of the organization, but to the user or, in our case, the patient:

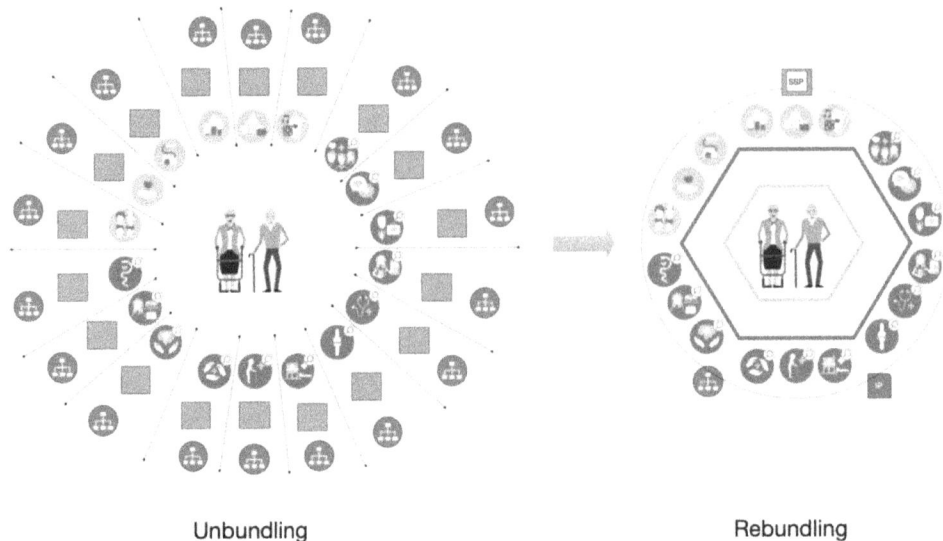

Unbundling   Rebundling

Figure 6.8 – Unbundling and rebundling healthcare organizations

This is all about the patient's **health experience** or **HeX**. Care organizations that adopt Rendanheyi would be better equipped to listen directly to the patients and provide care regarding the exact needs of the patient. The organization is unbundled into micro-enterprises and then rebundled into ecosystem micro-communities for customer-focused operations, demolishing existing silos in the organization. The organizational silos are demolished, so to speak, and the care teams are enabled by the **shared service platform** (**SSP**) with shared resourcing, which is governed by the **industry platform** (**IP**).

How can we put this in the ecocycle pattern? Each development stage can follow the **platform design toolkit** (**PDT**) phases and **Entrepreneurial Ecosystem Enabling Organization** (**EEEO**) toolkit from Boundaryless.io to achieve this value with the following:

- Exploration
- Strategic design
- Validation and prototyping
- Growth hacking

Without going into detail now, the takeaway from this approach is to concentrate on customer value and not fixed procedures or guidelines. In *Chapter 9, Working with Complex (System of) Systems, Chapter 10, Assessments with TiSH,* and *Chapter 11, Planning, Designing, and Architecting the Transformation,* we will dive into micro-enterprises and ecosystem micro-communities in more detail.

We can plot the platform design phases in the ecocycle to organize micro-enterprises, as shown in the following diagram:

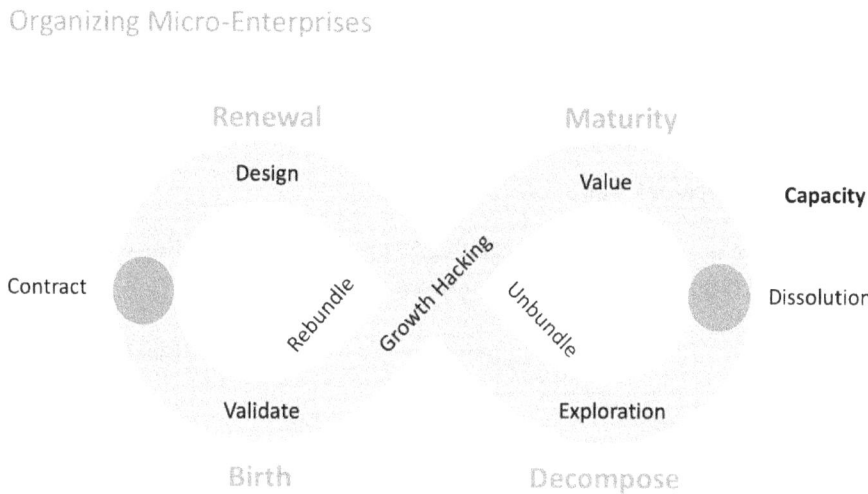

Figure 6.9 – The ecocycle for organizing micro-enterprises

The value at the organizational level is in creating enough capacity in micro-enterprises to provide healthcare required by the patients. It's the capacity to deliver that creates revenue. The panarchy connections, as put forward in *Figure 6.3*, are that in the Exploration stage, the organization can inspire the upstairs networked care treads to consider letting go and get involved and accelerate transition because capacity is available. On the other hand, if no added value is recognized, this will lead to the inhibition to contract the organization to build the capacity for delivering the new networked care. This transformation can be accelerated by organizing common understanding in HeX sessions so that more focus is put on the patient and how to optimize the value in the care network with a platform.

The challenge now is how to transition to the next networked treads, as shown in *Figure 6.10* in the next section. After all, the team of teams and organizations need to adapt to these forms of networked care. We can do this by following the unbundling and rebundling cycles, as per the networked care type:

- From unbundling traditional hierarchical structures in organizations to rebundling virtually in connected organizations for ad hoc networks around patients. The organizations know of each other's actions. They are visible to each other.

- Rebundling again via teams collaborating and forming the HeXagon by understanding each other regarding why they are involved in the network and coordinating accordingly in a formalized way.

- Using the acknowledged platform that supports the HeXagon to plan what has to happen in the integrated care plan.

- Building the ecosystems for directed care in the HeXagon to jointly determine the best cause of action.

The panarchy connections explore new ways to utilize the platform and trigger upstairs and being of value as a prerequisite to downstairs getting contracted.

Defining the care network ecocycle

We can define the care network ecocycle by getting a common understanding of respective case management, stepped care, integrated care, and directed care models:

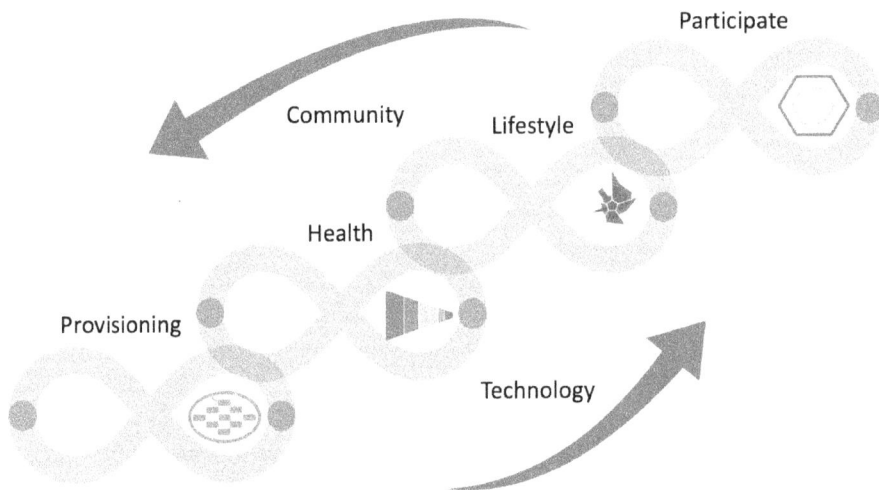

Figure 6.10 – The care network ecocycle

The platform consists of the technology that triggers the acceleration and the community that decelerates to determine the value before applying the platform. Both forces are essential to driving the transformation.

From the perspective of teams, they can experience the evolution toward a true ecosystem while still in the **claws** of the hierarchy, then the loosely forming virtual network around the patient and the serious steps of the team of teams and the platform, and finally, the ecosystem.

> **Note**
>
> To understand the developmental stages of networks, the works of David Ronfeldt are insightful. His **TIMN** model stands for **Tribal (kinship), Institution (hierarchy), Market (competition), and Network (connection)**.

It's the willingness to let go of the hierarchy that prepares the ground for unbundling. The lack of value seems to be the most obvious reason for the dilemma. Therefore, asking what true value we will deliver to patients and people is what leads to reasoning in how value is added to the ultimate outlook on participation. As Stowe Boyd writes:

That's why we are transitioning to platforms that support ecosystems, and the organizational form best suited to this is the "team of teams" model, such as Rendanheyi. Platform ecosystems will favor the team of teams organizational model for the participating companies.

(https://medium.com/work-futures/evolution-of-the-platform-organization-3-haier-rendanheyi-and-zhang-ruimins-vision-d8afceef7f5e)

Now that we have built our panarchy and established the interaction between the ecocycles, it's time to learn how the task force addresses the inhibition points. Therefore, we have to go back to people again. It's their state of mind that will determine how the transitions take place. Can we identify certain archetypes of behavior in change and can we look at this at the group level to understand why an individual, team, organization, or care network is at that point in their ecocycle?

Understanding people's states of mind

In the previous section, we discussed two main movements in transformation: technology-driven acceleration and community deceleration or inhibition. Simply put, technology is developing faster than the community is accepting and capable of adopting new technology. Often, this is explained by the *fear* of that new technology, but that's rarely true. The issue is that people are not trained to use the technology properly or they are not convinced of the added value. This is probably the main reason developers have a poor understanding of the real needs. The latter is typically fed by perception. Misperception or *myths* lead to inhibition, especially since one of the characteristics of societies is solidarity and protecting other people. Myths are widely spread and often rigidly fixed, reinforcing inhibition. Only some disruption will break this force. This force is called *understanding customer needs*. With this force, DevOps can create real value.

How do we overcome inhibition by understanding the needs of the people involved? Let's present some widely used transformation models to understand their stories and behaviors: Lippitt-Knoster, Rogers, Moore, and the already explained Mezirow. The Lippitt-Knoster model might be a good tool to start with since it describes the emotions of the people involved. This is very useful in our human-centric approach. Lippitt-Knoster describes the various *ingredients* to make a complex transformation successful. This model is shown in the following diagram:

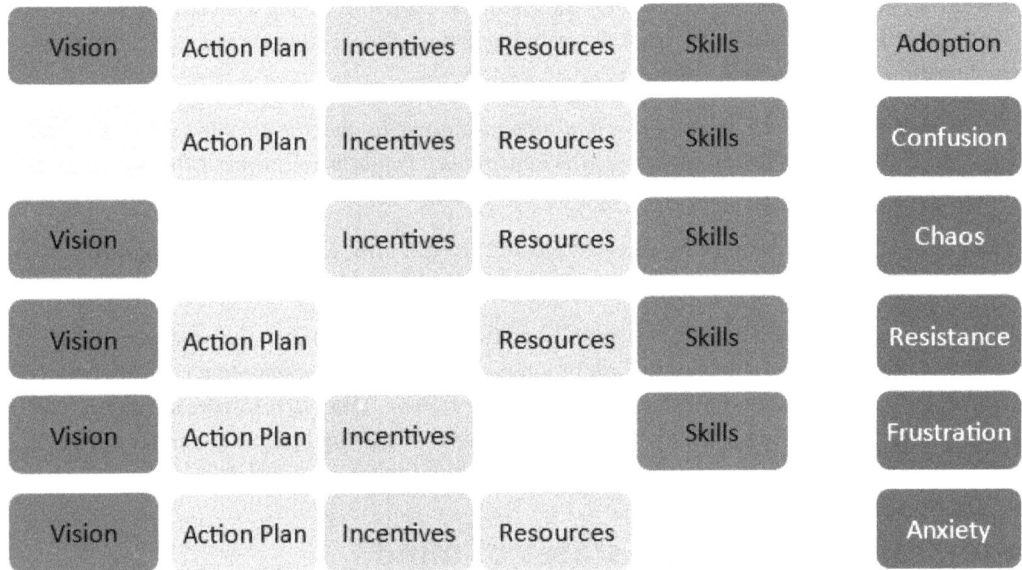

Vision	Action Plan	Incentives	Resources	Skills	Adoption
	Action Plan	Incentives	Resources	Skills	Confusion
Vision		Incentives	Resources	Skills	Chaos
Vision	Action Plan		Resources	Skills	Resistance
Vision	Action Plan	Incentives		Skills	Frustration
Vision	Action Plan	Incentives	Resources		Anxiety

Figure 6.11 – The Lippitt-Knoster model for Managing Complex Change

Next to the formal ingredients is the need to create change and transformation, which also addresses the emotions associated with change. This can be very helpful when exploring ideas and designs. As architects, we must take the following steps:

1. Start with a **Vision** and an **Action Plan** (through mission, goals, and strategy). This prevents false starts and **Confusion**.

2. Make sure that the (digital) **Resources** are working perfectly together, including the support of these resources. The users must be encouraged to develop their **Skills** while addressing **Anxiety** and **Frustration**.

3. Make sure **Incentives** are in place (create personal actionable urgency) and avoid anticipated **Resistance**.

It should be clear that behavior is an essential, if not the most important, element in transformation in each tread, especially in the speed at which innovation is or has to be adopted. There has to be a clear incentive or urgency. If a project is not giving the expected functionality and support, the transformation stops here with a lot of frustration and anxiety. This is the fundamental challenge for the architect: they need to find a solution for this. At the very least, they must be able to understand the consultants and medical staff regarding what the requirements must be. However, architects should also have an understanding of how users will respond to the introduction and adoption of innovative solutions. The architect can use this to define the incentive to get to faster adoption. Again, the digicoaches, e-nurses, and lead users play an important role in this.

Another well-known model is the Rogers adoption curve, which divides any group into five distinct types of behavior. Combined with Lippitt-Knoster, you can get an indication of who will be the first and last to adapt to a new way of digital working. An innovator only requires some skills to participate to overcome anxiety. Early adopters are typically satisfied if the technology is working and can avoid frustration. They are the typical lead users:

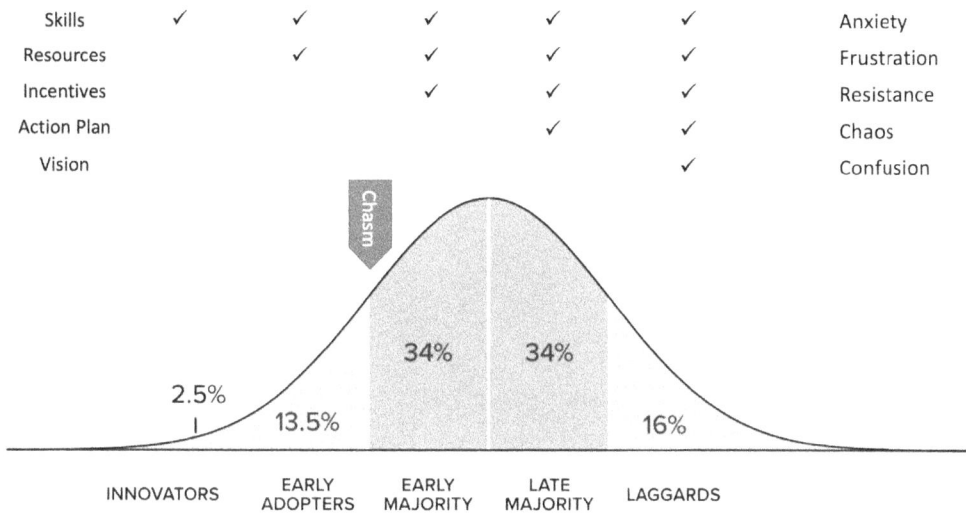

Figure 6.12 – The Lippitt-Knoster model combined with Rogers' adoption curve and Moore's chasm

In our transformation, we will be adopting new technology to provide care, but to make that a success, we need care providers to be trained in the use of this technology. That's where the digicoaches come in – professionals that will guide other care providers in adopting the new technology, mostly by learning that this will lead to better outcomes and eventually a better outlook for the patient. This process will follow the adoption curve, as recognized by Rogers. This curve shows the distribution of perceived risk and subsequent emotions and risk avoidance of people. More perceived risk means a longer time to adapt.

A notorious inhibition point is between the early adaptors and early majority, as described by Moore in *Crossing the Chasm*. We will come across him again in this book.

In other words, adopting new technology and innovations might be more about behavior than about acquiring (technical) skills, which is the playing field of e-nurses. Make no mistake: the technical skills must be trained too, but it starts with adoption. This is where the following steps take place:

1. Use the innovators in the DevOps team, and initially in the start-up phase.

2. Use the early adopters as lead users and contact the users in the scale-up phase.

3. In the scale-up phase, members of the early majority are instrumental in getting user feedback about their role as digicoaches, which is supported by floor walkers from IT and e-nurses.

Here, we can see the importance of including these roles in our TEC teams. Lead users, digicoaches, and e-nurses (or other medical roles) are crucial to letting the teams adapt quickly to new technologies. Moreover, we can think of these roles as the driving forces in adapting and accepting the technology itself.

If we combine Lippitt-Knoster and Rogers/Moore, we can define the ecocycle to start understanding behavior in transformation. This is the essence of shared mental models – assessing on what level we are, agreeing upon that, and deciding where we want to go:

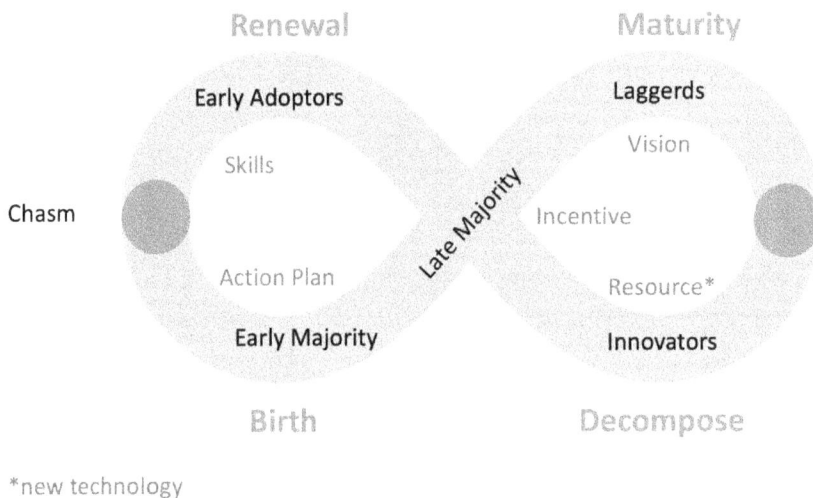

Figure 6.13 – Ecocycle combining Lippitt-Knoster and Rogers/Moore

The preceding figure shows that only involving innovators and early adaptors will not lead to success. However, new technology can trigger an innovator to come up with ideas. Early adopters can take this idea further once they master the necessary skills. An action plan should be available to overcome the chasm. The late majority and laggards are the people who mostly look at the achieved value and not the technology itself. Therefore, their stories are very valuable indeed.

While listening to these stories, ensure that you get a balanced view of the different people and their state of risk avoidance, learning, and circumstances, for health professionals as patients and next of kin alike. Otherwise, you end up jumping to the wrong conclusions and solutions.

Also, be aware of the Dunning-Kruger effect, in which people (individual treads) tend to overestimate the short-term value of technology and underestimate the long-term value. This makes it difficult to estimate when technology will be adopted at scale. Sometimes, this is called the **VUCA** world, which stands for **Volatile, Uncertain, Complex, and Ambiguous**. The best remedy we can think of for now is involving the lead users, digicoaches, and e-nurses. They should have a good grasp of the required needs.

By knowing when and how to listen to stories, given the state of mind of the storytellers, we can see the added value of community builders. Where can you find them? Like systems engineers have their INCOSE community, the community builders also have communities. One of them is known as Systems Innovation or Si Network (`https://www.systemsinnovation.network/feed`). They are an online collaborative platform for systems thinking and systems change. They work to empower the diversity of individuals and organizations in learning and applying systems innovation ideas and methods toward tackling complex challenges. This also applies to the healthcare sector and helps medical staff, management, and engineers.

Before starting the transformation, be sure that the task force taps into this community.

Summary

We have to agree on a common goal and a model for how to reach that goal. The challenge is that circumstances constantly change at different speeds. This is what panarchy is about: it describes how economic growth and human development interact and depend on ecosystems. In this chapter, we applied the principles of panarchy to the development of healthcare using ecocycle planning. These ecocycles help us take the subsequent steps on our TiSH journey.

The challenge in any transformation is that events happen at different speeds. We used the example of adopting technology: introducing a new technology happens faster than how individuals, teams, and organizations can adopt the new technology. Adoption requires planning to help us get where we want to be as an individual, team, organization, or network.

We also learned about inhibition: we can have technological acceleration, but there will be forces that cause inhibition and decelerate the adoption of technology. There must be something in it for individual professionals and, ultimately, for teams and organizations to start adoption. It has to fit their state of mind, both individually and in groups. We looked at the Lippitt-Knoster model for Managing Complex Change and the Rogers adoption curve, which showed that we need to include new roles in healthcare such as digicoaches and e-nurses to become early adopters. They will tell the stories that will feed DevOps.

All this requires a shared understanding of the goals and objectives and the agreed-upon structures that our healthcare teams will work with. Organizing common understanding activities when people are in the right state of mind is the way for the transformation task force to accelerate the transformation and build shared mental models.

In the next chapter, we will build further on these shared mental models.

Further reading

To learn more about the topics that were covered in this chapter, take a look at the following resources:

- *Panarchy: Understanding Transformations in Human and Natural Systems*, by L. Gunderson and C.S. Holling, 2001

- *Evolution of the Platform Organization*, by Stowe Boyd, Work Future at `https://www.workfutures.io`

- *Systems Innovation Toolbox* at `https://www.systemsinnovation.network/topics/7192272`

7
Creating New Platforms with OODA

As our knowledge and experience grow, we see patterns emerging. A MoM TiSH will now introduce us to **Observe-Orient-Decide-Act (OODA)**.

You are halfway through this book. The first half consisted of breaking down the complexity of transformation into most of the building blocks of TiSH. Now, we can start composing the transformation from the bottom up, filling in the blanks, and designing the enabling platform. When we think of *platforms*, we need a common ground – a shared mental model – on which to build new healthcare structures in a community. In this chapter, we will explore the main shared mental model, OODA, as the foundation of a healthcare transformation enabled by technology.

We will elaborate on OODA as a novel way to drive transformation with its feedback loops. In this chapter, the building blocks from TiSH will be put to use in the transformation of sustainable healthcare by creating disruptive platforms that enable teams to dynamically plan resources around a patient.

In the final part of the chapter, we will learn what the transformations made to these platforms look like and how they can be shaped. As an example, we will analyze Amazon Care, Buurtzorg, and Roamler Care as recent initiatives in transforming healthcare.

In this chapter, we're going to cover the following topics:

- Understanding and applying the building blocks
- Applying OODA feedback loops to create transformative platforms
- Analyzing platform-driven transformation

Understanding and applying the building blocks

As a transformation task force, we know we have to bridge the three perspectives of provisioning healthcare, enabling the community, and implementing technology platforms with a shared mental model that is understood by medical or social staff, community builders, and systems engineers.

In *Figure 5.10* of *Chapter 5, Leveraging TiSH as Toolkit for Common Understanding*, we presented the building blocks of the TiSH value stairway with some blanks still to fill in. In this chapter, we discuss how OODA will form the principle-of shared mental model to integrate these building blocks. In later chapters, we will use the OODA shared mental model for a common understanding to define the blanks and integrate the building blocks into TiSH.

Let's start creating the OODA shared mental model. In the following figure, we can see the building blocks arranged around OODA:

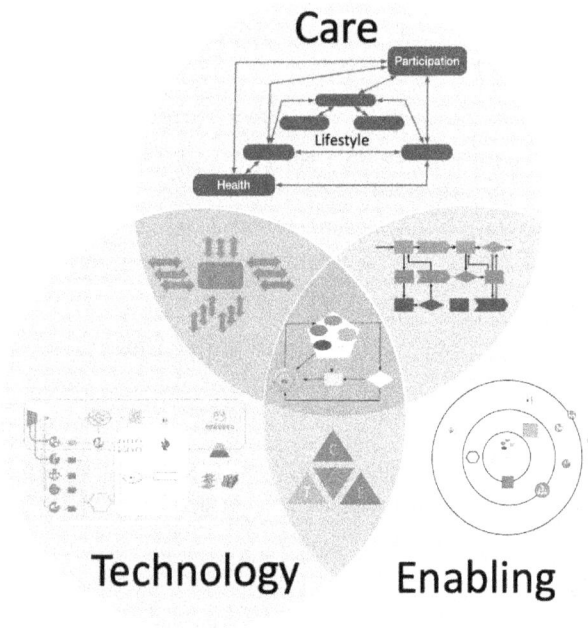

Figure 7.1 – OODA's central shared mental model

Each of the building blocks is related to OODA. Care provisioning is observing a person's life in terms of health, lifestyle, and participation and orienting continuously to decide what actions to take to either anticipate, prevent, or cure an illness. It works in accordance with the workflows of enabling the community and interacting with a technology platform.

Enabling community, organized to provide and support micro-enterprises within ecosystem micro-communities, defines the workflows and supports the OODA processes in accordance with the activity triangle to safeguard the human element and perspective.

The technology platform makes the OODA functions available and interactive, supports care provisioning, and is designed in the context of the activity triangle.

Now, we will discuss the perspective of care provisioning, enabling community, and the technology platform a bit further.

Reacting to health, lifestyle, and participation events with OODA

We discussed the OODA loop extensively in *Chapter 4*, *Including the Human Factor in Transformation*, but it's good to shortly recap the principles.

In essence, OODA describes how an individual observes a situation based on the available data. All decisions are based on observations. The OODA loop shows observations coming from unfolding circumstances and interactions. These observations lead to information that is processed in the orient phase.

In other words, observations do not immediately lead to decisions and actions. Observations are filtered through human factors: experiential, cultural, and heritage, such as the quality assurance system of a care organization. The enriched information will eventually lead to decision-making and action. That decision leads to new events and that will lead to new observations and eventually, reactions or proactive anticipation.

To speed up the reaction time and reach better, more accurate outcomes, we must implement the OODA loop in the health journey of the patient or patient population to prevent worsening health conditions and detect early symptoms. Different circumstances and interactions unfold in terms of health, lifestyle, and participation. For the care provider to be in control of the situation, the changeable state of health, health conditions, and personal circumstances need to be continually observed. As we have seen in *Chapter 4*, *Including the Human Factor in Transformation*, this requires accurate data on the events that unfold.

However, this data is not readily available. It takes a lot of effort to get the data. For a better understanding, we look at the status of digitization in care provisioning from an OODA perspective. On the left-hand side of *Figure 2.3*, the typical activities mentioned were presented in *Chapter 2, Exploring Relevant Technologies for Healthcare*. On the right-hand side are the characteristics of this type of networked care:

OODA steps	Digital Provisioning (Treatment, therapy, or intervention)
	(Ad hoc network communication)
Act data on: Self- or case management Intake Preparation Multidisciplinary provisioning	Actions are registered in terms of type, time, and material for management purposes, such as planning, salary payments, purchasing, and logistics related to materials – typically, the functionality found in the **Enterprise Resource Planning** (**ERP**) systems. Emphasis on how things are going to be done with what resources for the internal organization and externally for other organizations in the ad hoc network – whatever has been done is communicated.
Decide data on: Shared decision-making	Decisions on therapy, such as starting, stopping, or adapting an intervention. Classified in terms of the **International Classification of Functioning, Disability, and Health** (**ICF**) **model** – for example: not able to walk (activity) due to knee injury (body function), logged in a digital system. This type of data is, among others, used for reimbursement and billing in the financial system. Emphasis on why you are acting for external accountability reasons.
Orient data on: Diagnostics/self-diagnostics	The triage, assessment, and diagnostics are registered typically in the **Electronics Patient Record** (**EPR**). This can be based on narrative, structured, or standardized (coded) in terms of the ICF model or another medical model. This substantive information on the initial assessment is used for healthcare provisioning. Emphasis on what to do within the cultural and inherited context (protocols) and based on the analysis of previous experience (recorded digitally) and new information from observation.
Observe data on: Circumstances Assessment Observe outcome	The digital registration of observations such as tests, as in, blood tests, CT scans in lab systems, or **Picture Archiving and Communication Systems** (**PACSs**). Observations can also be communicated by other care providers as part of a referral. Equally, the push button of a social alarm system or a sensor with movement detection are examples of digitized observations. They all provide new information for the Orient step. It's this step where more and more emphasis on digital information collection creates opportunities for transformation due to advances in technology, such as smart watches and implants.

Table 7.1 – OODA steps in digital provisioning

Each of the activities exchanges its observation, orientation, decision, or actions with other activities carried out by team members or teams – either within a healthcare organization or between organizations. Think of a GP deciding to prescribe medication that will be delivered by the pharmacist. In this rudimentary ad hoc networked care, communication is required.

With people following workflows in the systems, as mentioned here, whether ERP, EPRs, sensors from alarm buttons, or PACSs, these workflows can be integrated to form automated OODA loops. This integration via workflows is required to enable team members to interact seamlessly with the platform and be more focused on their primary job, care provisioning to patients. The care work activities are integrated to guide the patient through their health journey.

If we apply OODA to formal (not ad hoc), networked care, new opportunities arise, as described in the following table:

OODA loops	Digital provisioning (Treatment, therapy, or Intervention)
Joint Observe loop: Stepped care Collaborate Coordinate	Provide therapy until the target has been met or the therapy needs to be stepped up or down. To know whether therapy has been effective, observation of the developments or changes to health conditions and circumstances are required to determine when to act by stepping up, stepping down, or stopping therapy. This requires constant logging and (real- or near real-time) processing of the events, acting following the implicit guidance of the stepped care guidelines, and transferring the therapy to the right step. This is not a complete OODA loop but a joint Observe-Orient loop. Decisions and actions are within a single team or organization as part of the collaboration. Social alarms are a good example of a shortcut observation loop. When an alarm goes off, it raises awareness that something may be going on and a decision is made to gauge via smart speakers, such as Amazon Echo, Google Home, or Apple HomePod, whether something severe has happened, such as an injury occurring, and whether to act by sending a nurse to attend. The nurse can send the patient to a GP or hospital if needed. Further on, we will see this requires a good amount of digital service management. The focus is on health conditions such as COPD (Chronic Obstructive Pulmonary Disease), as with the Nearklinikken in Denmark.
Joint Diagnostics loop: Integrated care Acknowledged cooperation Control	During integrated care, reassessing the initial diagnostics is continual, with repeated measurement of specific conditions and target activities or behavior. Having data available before, during, and after an intervention allows for trend analysis, the analysis of changes in conditions, or of behavior that was targeted by lifestyle-related therapy. New diagnostics can ascertain that lifestyle intervention needs to be continued by some other team. This can mean referral within the acknowledged cooperation of integrated care networks to switch the target set – for instance, from psychology therapy for anxiety control to stopping smoking (as a habit) as a target. Strictly, the Action element occurs within separate teams, but observation of the patient, orientation, and decision-making are all done jointly. The focus is on the lifestyle of patients with comorbidity problems and preventing episodes related to one or more health conditions as much as possible.

Joint Treatment loop:	The final step is that the loop overarches all treatments or interventions to improve health conditions and overall lifestyle with directed care's goal of participation in mind. Once an event is detected (or observed), it requires an intervention (an adjustment). Think of quantified self-monitoring and extensive monitoring of external conditions, such as air quality, weather, or pollen in the air.
Directed care	Although this loop can be performed within one organization, it will certainly involve different teams, which have to communicate and make shared decisions.
Direct	Here, observation is focused on the ability to participate. It requires a continuous assessment based on observations and (digitally) adjusted treatment. Occupational healthcare is a relevant area. What treatments allow you to be able to perform your job optimally and prevent occupational hazards? Another example is when the weather forecast predicts icy roads and walkways and issues an alert to elderly people to wear their hip airbags so they can safely go outdoors.
Command	This is a complete joint OODA loop, with the Action also incorporated in the joint operations.
	However, be aware that not everything can be measured and digitized. That's why it's good to keep a human in the loop.

Table 7.2 – OODA loops in digital provisioning

With a common understanding from a medical perspective, OODA can be translated for healthcare provisioning and applied to the processes and workflows used by care and support teams.

Enabling the OODA activities

To enable the care teams, fitting workflows to their activities is required – workflows to connect the OODA steps within the organization and jointly within teams in different types of networked care. Communication workflows, coordination workflows, control workflows, and command workflows enable the patient-facing ecosystem and micro-community to work together.

The following table describes the combination of network type and type of workflows for each OODA step:

Observe	Observe the actions of others involved in the ad hoc network	Jointly observe health	Jointly observe lifestyle	Jointly observe outlook on participation
Orient	Internal orientation on each activity	Conditional notification for referral in accordance with the guidelines on collaboration	Multi-disciplinary orientation	Jointly orient on what intervention to take, fusing observations and simulating the consequences
Decide	Internal decisions on each activity	Notification of a specific step to coordinate the transfer	Joint decision on which interventions to provide, controlled by lifestyle targets	The individual directs the outlook on participation – for example, in terms of mobility Decisions on which intervention to choose, supporting the outlook
Act	Internal actions are executed independently and communicated to other teams or organizations	Communicate health problem-related information	An integral plan for the care providers is made related to lifestyle and independently but cooperatively executed	Full cooperation focused on participation and commands to teams or devices, to deliver information and interventions accordingly
OODA Network				

Table 7.3 – The stages of digitization

Community builders will focus on the OODA loops related to communication, collaboration, coordination, control, command, and cooperation in the care networks.

With the workflows agreed on, we will now have a look at the information we need.

Data processing on the technology platform

How do we get data that gives us an accurate view of events and recognizes patterns, thus leading to appropriate responses? To answer that question, we first need to ask: what is an event and how can we make it digital so that it can be communicated to anyone in the care network?

An event is anything that causes a significant change to somebody's health condition, lifestyle, participation, or circumstances. These events are, in principle, observable and therefore convertible into digital information. The following diagram shows how the event is observed by collecting data and processing this data to lead to a decision or action as output. This output forms new information that's looped back to the condition or circumstances of the patient:

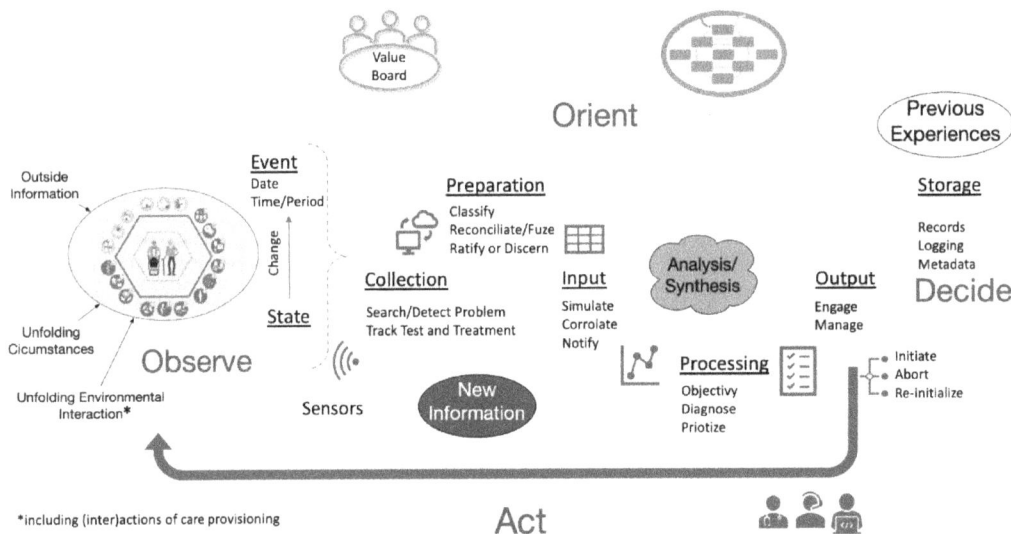

Figure 7.2 – Data processing with the OODA loop

Events create data that we can observe. The collection of the data can be done by the patient entering an event into a website or by a doctor – a GP, for example – entering the data following medical protocols. The patient can be observed using sensors, check-ups, specific tests, and diagnostics, but also by events that are reported by the patient or by social networks surrounding the patient noticing an event. To recap, we can define an event as anything that causes a significant change to a health condition or personal circumstances.

If the data and therefore the observations lead to any concerns, then orientation starts: why is the event happening, or why did it? From this point onward, it gets interesting. The typical decision or action is to admit the patient to a clinical pathway with fixed workflows and processes. The pathway is bundled, so to speak. In the traditional way of providing healthcare, this is more or less a fixed journey for the patient, delivered from a hospital or other clinical organizations as one entity. This will be different in networked care.

We will analyze the data processing OODA loop depicted step by step. It's a combination of the elements of the OODA loop and **Machine Learning** (**ML**) data processing.

The collection of data involves observing the patient and their circumstances. Actors who are observing the patient are the following:

- The patient themselves (self-assessment)
- Social networks or next of kin
- Sensor equipment
- Check-ups
- Specific tests and diagnostics
- Environmental conditions

We can automate data collection and processing, but we need learning systems for this to achieve our transformation goals. That's where **Artificial Intelligence (AI)** with ML and digital twins will play a significant role. These technologies can tap into a vast repository of medical protocols and research data to create an ever faster learning loop to drive the transformation.

The end goal for the transformation is directed care where a personal case manager guides the patient through the agile clinical pathways. We foresee a development where the personal case manager as part of directed care will be an autonomous assistant based on current assistant technology, such as Siri, Google Assistant, Google Home, or Alexa.

The platform will evolve over time from tread to tread, driven by DevOps. With the aforementioned data processing model, the systems engineer has a simple but effective shared mental model to which they can relate the stories told by the care professionals.

Now, we, together with the systems engineers, must design the digital systems – the platform – that enable all this. We will discuss that in the following section.

Applying OODA feedback loops to create transformative platforms

We have learned that OODA is our shared mental model for looking at medical processes and how the activities of the enabling teams in micro-enterprises are executed and connected via workflows. We also learned how data processing can be mapped using OODA. Together, they provide the structure for the stories to be told as input for DevOps. However, remember *Chapter 6, Applying the Panarchy Principle*, to take the state of mind into account, and the use of CAFCR and QFD development methods, as explained in *Chapter 5, Leveraging TiSH as Toolkit for Common Understanding*.

Having said that, DevOps translates these stories into modular microservice architectures and shared platforms, as already common in IT. With the use of modern cloud functionality, organizations can plan resources dynamically: they use the resources when needed and only pay for these resources when they are used. If resources are no longer required, they are scaled down or suspended.

That's not something that you can do easily with big, monolithic, legacy systems. We would need to stop the entire system, where we still might want to use some of the services that these systems provide. If we require a new feature, we would need to upgrade the whole system and might even need to plan for significant downtime for testing to check whether a new feature disrupts the system. This does not lead to the agility to form dynamic care networks in collaborations and cooperations.

Explaining microservices

It's good to explain what microservices are all about. In contradiction to monolithic systems that are designed as one piece, microservices are loosely coupled components that form a system. You will recognize the bundling and rebundling principle here: the big monolith is transformed into a system that consists of loosely coupled modular components. The problem with monolithic systems is that they slow down innovation since it's very hard to adopt changes within these systems. The significant advantage of microservices is that systems become more agile and scalable to swiftly accommodate the new workflows in networked care and are an important prerequisite to making the systems more modular.

As a matter of fact, it's very hard to react to events and apply changes accordingly in vast, legacy systems. That's the reason we need to unbundle monolithic systems and rebundle them into modular microservices systems so that they can be rapidly reconfigured for the required care networks.

In our case, the OODA microservices need to be interacted with using easy **user interfaces** (**UXs**) and stimulate individuals to do their work, but there's also a major risk that we must consider. If more and more systems are integrated to cope with the interactions between teams, organizations, and care networks, resulting in activities with ever more types of stimuli, simultaneously in ever broader environments, it can very easily lead to an overload of stimuli from the other systems. **Robotic Process Automation** (**RPA**) and AI are required to cope with this increasing complexity without overloading individuals.

The systems engineers are tasked with designing the technological platform with intuitive systems of engagement. On the one hand, we see many great opportunities in things such as big data, ML, AI, and bioengineering, but we also see the potential undesirable effects these can have on people and, more generally, society. Patients, care providers, organizations, and society at large need time to digest the new possibilities before taking well-founded decisions. The consequences can be profound. Remember the de-decelerating forces in the panarchy.

Alongside microservices, it is at the level of these individual components that interoperability must be built in to enable integration at higher levels. With this in mind, we can start the design of the microservices. Therefore, we use the following five categories of components in systems:

- Actors such as people and machines as effectors in the physical world or performers of data processing, requiring a system of engagement.

- Sensors translating events and stimuli, whether these are people observing events and registering them in a digital system, simple detectors, such as a motion detector, or complex sensors, such as an MRI scanner or ML detecting a pattern in data. The latter includes algorithms analyzing real-time vital signs or smartwatches sensing a fall. These require systems of recording and systems of intelligence.

- Controllers for managing the activities and workflows, including when to take decisions in processes, either manually made on the part of humans or software-automated, also requiring systems of intelligence.

- Stimuli, as in, external and observable events and triggers between entities of sensors, controllers, and actors. This can range from a simple notification of a personal alarm to large amounts of data, such as 4D CT or MRI scans. These stimuli come typically from the Internet of Things.

- The environment, which influences the performance of the functions – for example, the conditions in which entities can perform. An MRI scanner typically needs a well-equipped hospital to function. A wearable gives more freedom but has fewer capabilities. Typical environments are hospitals, nursing homes, practices, homes, workplaces, outdoors, or transport. The environment is part of the system too.

The systems engineers have to explore possible solutions in (re)designing monolithic systems into modular microservices together with the users and other stakeholders, such as the community builders. The OODA functions and these system components plotted along the healthcare activities are the structures used to explore options and tell stories in healthcare. Not the underlying technologies.

Nevertheless, how do we transform from the current often monolithic systems to the new microservices?

Reversed build of the OODA loop

Can you imagine a hospital letting go of its buildings and each room in it, including all the equipment and staff? Next, staff and equipment are micro-rented by the dedicated teams around a patient. This could be done if we developed platforms and systems as microservices and had micro-enterprises as care teams. Food for thought, at least for now.

The message is that if we want to transform healthcare, we must let go of traditional thinking and of doing things simply because we have learned to do it in a specific way. That's why we build on the principles of the OODA loop in order to facilitate the transition.

We must address OODA functions such as Act by selecting the required components, whether actors, sensors, or controllers, and determining the stimuli to which they need to respond (input) or that they need to provide (output) and which individuals will be using it in the environment. These individuals can be machines or devices, care professionals, supporting staff, or people to whom care is provided.

Actors perform a single task or multiple activities in a workflow as part of a process that the microservice supports.

Before they can act, the environment, including the required equipment, must be prepared. If a device is not already installed, it needs to be ordered and installed in such a way that it's integrated into the workflow and operational for the individuals involved. This requires a professionally managed device service or services that includes support for the end user, the care professional, and the patient alike.

> **Note**
>
> This is not solely about the big irons such as CT and MR scanners but is also true for a device that takes an **electrocardiogram** (**ECG**) of the patient at home. The device needs to be set up for the patient. It's even true for something as simple as a personal alarm system or medicine dispenser. It needs to be installed and configured so that it can support the patient in the proper way. Before the act of actually dispensing medicine, other actions already have taken place. It's applicable to almost every action, including installing apps for self-help.

Microservices can be designed and built for each of the components for the OODA functions. Interoperability between these microservices is a design requirement for forming the OODA loops.

We have unbundled the systems into the related components at the task and activity level for each OODA step and are able to rebundle them into the required loop. At this stage, it's important to keep track of the configuration and relations of each of the many components in terms of interoperability. For a micro-services approach to succeed, an **Application Programming Interface** (**API**) strategy is required. Legacy systems can also be gradually replaced with microservices in this way.

The significant benefit is that we now have the foundation for agile iterative innovation and transformation.

Now, go back to *Table 7.2* and *Table 7.3*. Here, the four OODA steps and three OODA loops were related to the healthcare activities and the current ERP and EPR systems used in those activities.

We propose to (re)build the legacy systems into microservices recycling the same sequence, which is reversed from OODA to ADOO, so to speak:

- **Act**: Define the components with the required interoperability characteristics to communicate between activities, both inside and outside the organization

- **Decide**: Integrate decision-making for the teams, taking input from inside and outside the organization

- **Orient**: Facilitate the following in organizations:

  - Genetic heritage in guardrails, guidelines, and protocols, including formal decision points as agreed by law, in collaboration in stepped care or cooperation in integrated or directed care

  - Culture and traditions in mandates, processes, and intuitive workflow interactions in systems of engagement

  - Analytics or synthesis in algorithms in systems of intelligence

- Previous experiences with logging, storing, and retrieving records in systems

- New information acquired and data from sensors processed

- **Observations**: They become relevant when the patient and its network are involved by connecting their data to the activities of other organizations.

- **Observation loop**: Workflows for collaboration to coordinate each provisioning in stepped care

- **Diagnose loop**: Control workflows in integrated care

- **Treatment loop**: Command workflows in directed care

Following this sequence implies that time will be required for rebuilding. However, the sequence is purposely aligned with the TiSH staircase to keep technological and community change in sync.

In the next chapter, we will go into more detail. By defining the OODA loops, we have a way to explore the requirements and solutions for the enabling platform with the actual users.

Analyzing platform-driven transformation

In the previous sections, we discussed new systems for observing patients, driving decisions, and acting upon them. We talked about sensors and *observers* around the patient collecting data, allowing accurate diagnostics to be made by highly skilled practitioners and personal case management, assisted by simulations using ML and personalized medicine. These are all promising developments, but since we are discussing DevOps4Care, we must take Ops into careful consideration as well. Operations are critical in the delivery of end-to-end managed services for the sensors and other equipment, including apps and interfaces.

This is where models such as IT4IT come in. These models recognize the enabling platforms that must be managed and the product teams that develop and deploy the services on top of that platform. IT4IT uses value streams to identify and design the IT resources required to deliver end-to-end services based on the customer journey. In our case, that would be the journey of the patient and the actors in their network. New digital roles such as an e-nurse identify the needs – these are translated into services in a specialized team that makes use of microservices from managed platforms, allowing them to dynamically scale resources.

Clearly, this is not a transformation that is done overnight. We must follow the rules of DevOps and agile here. If we look at our TiSH staircase MoM, we must start with a **Minimal Viable Product (MVP)** at every tread: from there, development and deployment will be done step by step, taking inhibition points into account.

To succeed, organizations, teams, networks, and even societies on national levels need to be on the same page with shared mental models. Shared mental models, however, take time to build. Learning must be an integral part of the system on all levels. Otherwise, many unrelated and incompatible services (apps and programs) are not interoperable.

Therefore, we must build carefully on a step-by-step basis, starting with an MVP on each tread of our TiSH staircase.

Let's analyze some actual examples.

Amazon Care

Amazon Care started with its own employees to provide a fitting health experience via the app so that they were able to participate well in their work at Amazon. It's an MVP for directed care with the limited scope of, in this case, an ambulant nurse, e-doctor, and pharmacist. This covers most of the required medical attention and it provides a foundation for learning how to improve services and extend them to other groups. Learning is entrenched in the way of working, enabling Amazon Care to expand quickly. Amazon Care is as a next iteration offered to other employers in the US for their employees.

Buurtzorg

Buurtzorg has created a platform to support their specialized nurses to coordinate the care network around mostly elderly living independently at home. They create a stepped care approach for the inner (yellow) HeXagon, in which choices are made regarding what the client can do themselves, what their next of kin can do, and what can be done by the nurses at Buurtzorg. Specialized nurses are trained to oversee integral elderly care and know when to refer to other social or medical providers. This has proven to be very successful and has been adopted in many other countries.

Roamler Care

An example of an organization that has successfully implemented case management with a shared platform and executed unbundling and rebundling is Roamler Care. The organizations using Roamler Care's platform are unbundled in crowd-sourced communities and bundled via the platform, allowing for dynamic allocation of resources around a patient based on the ad hoc needs in the virtual network. It goes without saying that Roamler Care relies heavily on technology that enables the deployment of data-driven activities:

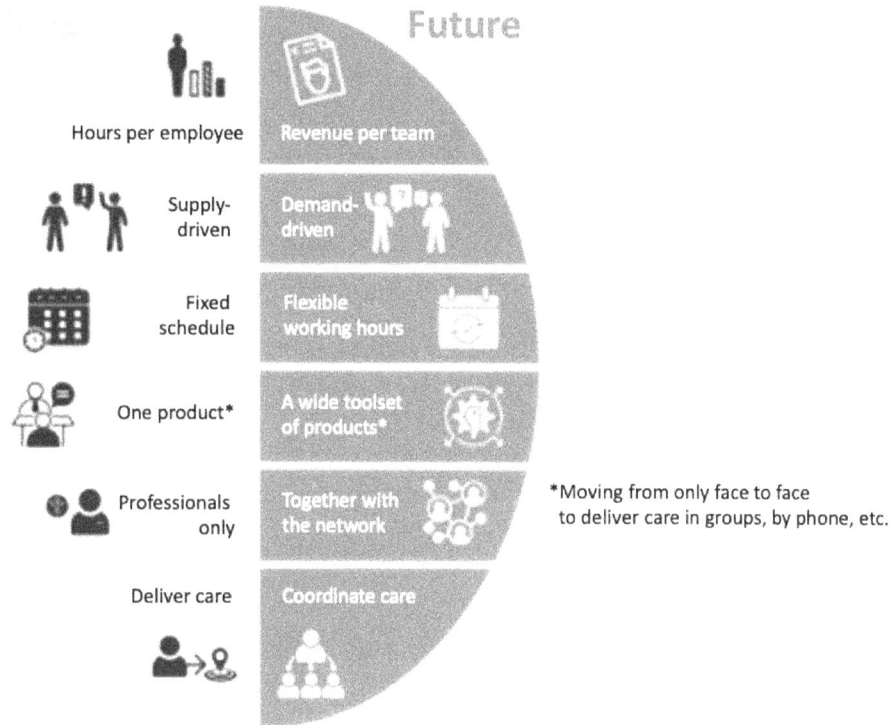

Figure 7.3 – Aspects of the transformation for Roamler

Roamler Care unbundles care in specific tasks, which leads to a more efficient allocation of resources. To enable this, Roamler Care works in a data-driven mode. The data is collected from millions of tasks performed annually by Roamler Care teams across Europe, allowing the organization to identify patterns and make predictions. It uses the data to streamline activities and organize resources better. Before applying this principle to healthcare, they use it for quality assurance in retail (as in, mystery shoppers) and to fulfill the installation of connected equipment, such as smart thermostats in homes via Roamler Tech.

How does Roamler Care collect that data? Via mobile technology that integrates with Roamler Care's own systems and other systems used by the professionals in the communities. In this way, care providers can work with independent care professionals and integrate them into their own organization in existing, permanent teams. It leverages the flexibility, scalability, and speed of activities at the right time, place, and for the right patient. Roamler Care provides the technology – the Roamler Care app, which is used to collect and show the tasks – and the management of the communities. It is the systems engineer and community builder.

> **Note**
>
> Roamler Care was founded in 2011 and has expanded to become an international organization with operations across Europe since then. More information can be found at `roamler.com`.

Organizations that work with Roamler Care stay in control through customer portals and dashboards. Obviously, data is protected and compliant with the defined and agreed guardrails.

Do you recognize all of the three examples from the previous sections in this chapter? You should since they are great examples of applying OODA design principles to platforms:

- Communication via care platform to enable case management to request resources when needed by Roamler
- Coordinate actions in a stepped care model by using an enabling platform, adhering to the principles of interoperability and integration by Buurtzorg
- Control via a platform by referring to the right provider for integral (elderly) care by Amazon and Buurtzorg
- Command directed by the patient based on their own health condition by Amazon

They all have joint quality control to build trust in the various networks and organizations and are learning to foster a customer-obsessed and collaborative approach to transforming healthcare and expanding this field.

Summary

In essence, this chapter was about events and how we can react to events. First, we explained what an event is: anything which causes a significant change in the health condition or personal circumstances. An event needs to be observed; we need to know that it happens. For that, we must collect data. In this chapter, we studied how we can collect and analyze the data, following the principles of OODA: Observe, Orient, Decide, and Act. We can use these principles to design our systems – that is, systems with the required feedback loops for both operational use and transformational learning.

In this chapter, we also learned how we can design systems by using microservices architectures. We have learned to unbundle and rebundle organizations – now, we must do the same with the systems that these organizations use. It's all about enabling the dynamic scaling of resources around the patient. We unbundle the tasks and the resources and provide these when and where the patient needs them. In the final section, we saw that this is not just theory: Amazon Care, Buurtzorg, and Roamler Care have unbundled and rebundled their organizations and made their systems flexible and scalable, responding to the needs of the patients.

We've studied the organization of healthcare and the future systems. In the following chapter, we will discuss how all of this works out for the actual teams and the health journeys of individuals.

Learning How Interaction Works in Technology-Enabled Care Teams

After education, it is time to work. MoM TiSH is sending us to the first job.

We studied the principles of shared mental models and applied these to design new platforms as a common ground for building sustainable healthcare – since that's what this book is all about. In the previous chapter, we elaborated on the **Observe-Orient-Decide-Act (OODA)** model as the main shared mental model, including the interaction between people, technology, and systems. A platform is more than just a collection of components; it's the interaction between the components and users that makes it come to life. We will learn all about these interactions in the health journey in this chapter.

We will discuss how the transformation task force can stimulate the community of care teams to share how they interact or want to interact with other actors in the healthcare ecosystem. We will do so by following the team and the activities throughout the health journey using the **Journey Interaction Matrix (JIM)**.

In this chapter, we're going to cover the following topics:

- Defining interactions in activities
- Shaping the journey for care teams and patients
- Exploring the roles of team members and patients

Defining interactions in activities

To get input for the platform development process, the Dev in DevOps, the task force organizes sessions to collect the stories from the potential users. The task force gives the care providers the opportunity to share what they need for their activities at certain touchpoints in the health journey.

For a common understanding, the OODA model is used. To get a structured story, we introduce the JIM. This is used to reason about the possibilities and formulate stories. These structured stories are used in the development process for the exploration of solutions and subsequent **Quality Functional Deployment** (**QFD**) and specifications, as explained in *Chapter 5, Leveraging TiSH as Toolkit for Common Understanding*.

Let's find out what the input for Dev is.

To achieve this, you could rely on generic metaphors, such as the village of blind people encountering an elephant and trying to describe it. However, it then still doesn't necessarily lead to the required shared understanding. The awareness of a specific situation itself is a good starting point for putting some effort into the storming phase of Tuckman's team development phases – we discussed Tuckman in *Chapter 5, Leveraging TiSH as Toolkit for Common Understanding*. The resulting understanding based on shared mental models is the norm to be able to perform.

In the previous chapter, we discussed the OODA principles for building system components and defining their interoperability and integration on each tread of our TiSH Staircase.

To avoid spending too much time in the storming phase in a team, you need a starting point for the process from which you can evolve into the norming phase. Formal models such as OODA can serve this purpose, as was our reasoning in the former chapter. At least, it jumpstarts the process of either using the models presented or rapidly finding other models that provide the required shared understanding for the problem to be solved.

In *Chapter 7, Creating New Platforms with OODA*, we brought forward the OODA principles for building system components, defining their interactions in terms of interoperability, and integrating on each tread. This will also be the central principle in this chapter on interactions between the activities of the **Technology-Enabled Care** (**TEC**) teams.

What we do is divide the activities into four categories, the OODA steps. On the user level, the interaction is in the activity and the interoperability and integration are between the activities.

In *Figure 8.1*, we find a very simple health journey to demonstrate. Observation consists of determining how much pain the patient is in. Next is to orient on what to do about the level of pain. If the pain affects behavior too much, then the pain killer dosage can be altered, resulting in giving a certain dose of medicine.

If in the orientation, the effect on behavior is not so much, then no action is needed, or it was time to give the medication anyway. These are the implicit guidance loops of OODA. No formal decision is required.

The lines between the OODA activities are significant for the enabling functions. The patient has to communicate their level of pain. A common way to do that is the **Visual Analog Scale** (**VAS**) or VAS score. It's a scale between 1 and 10. The behavior also has to be captured by video or text entry. Sending the information triggers orientation. If it is decided that the medicine should be altered, then this triggers an activity with the pharmacist:

Observe:
Pain

VAS score
Video

Orient:

**Effect on
behaviour**

Trigger decision-making

Decide:

**Altering
dose**

Take
medicine

Act:

**Give
medicine**

Change prescription and
deliver medicine

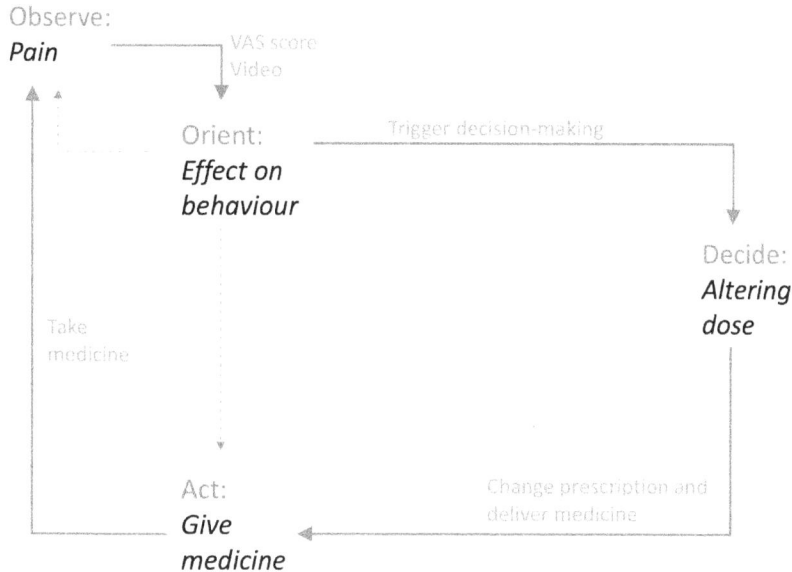

Figure 8.1 – OODA activities

We have learned how important it is to see these interactions in order to realize feedback loops. It starts with the availability of digital data in the first place if we want to make workflows in the enabling platform.

The challenge lies in the ever-increasing ways of observing and processing the acquired data and using that data in feedback loops.

There's a risk that we must consider in evangelizing digitization and that is that the possible overload and distraction on the actual job will lead to the inhibition of change. To avoid this, digital interactions must be intuitive and quick. If prior to interaction, the information has to be extracted from one or more systems in a cumbersome way and it takes (too much) time to prepare the data to be comprehensible and ready for interaction, then the data will probably be left unused.

Three are three major prerequisites to the use of data if we want to make an impact on workflow:

- Registration of data must be very easy and fault-free

- Accessibility or retrievability is quick and reliable with syntactic interoperability

- Comprehensible to sender and receiver with semantic interoperability

The data must be actionable – as in, consumable, believable, and usable for decision-making (the sender or receiver can take action on the data presented). There is no question about the authenticity, accuracy, or completeness of the data. The data must also be integrated into the workflow so that collection, transfer, and consumption are seamless and integrated into decision cycles. This requires not only digitization of the systems involved but also re-tooling of people through training and exposure and a rework of processes.

Shaping the journey for care teams and patients

The journey is one of continual health over a full lifetime. Already in *Chapter 2*, *Exploring Relevant Technologies for Healthcare*, we defined the **Health eXperience** (**HeX**) as the continuation of health and the services around it. These services optimize the HeX for as high a number of patients or clients that a care team can attend to as possible. Demand is driven in terms of improving health, lifestyle, and participation. This is done with flexible resources and a broad range of available technology-based support services. Services are coordinated within the ecosystem micro-communities. This requires activities and interactions between those activities.

With the OODA activities in mind, we need a way to structure the stories we get from the work floor. A structure derived from the HeX and health journeys, triggered by events in the health condition, is built on the interactions in the touchpoints within these journeys. We introduce the JIM that is presented in *Figure 8.2*, which can be used to define interactions along the journey. We use seven *W*-questions to define the journey:

- *Why is the journey needed?* What events led to the problem that has triggered a health assessment and defines the treatment and any associated care or health plan? There has to be a clear starting point in a journey to give meaning to the other questions. What are the goals in terms of health, lifestyle, and participation?

- *Who is taking part in the journey?* The patient is surrounded by many actors who are all concerned with the health of the patient. Think of informal caregivers (as in, next of kin or others in the social network), nurses, practitioners, or specialists from several care providers. Typically, procedures are confined or siloed in an organization, but we must take full advantage of all available resources around a person and what they can do with each other for this person.

- *What do they have to do; what is the purpose of an action or activity?* For example, exercising as part of the care or health plan or monitoring a heart condition. These are typically the medical protocols, procedures, and steps in related processes. Consider these to be the genetic heritage. These activities use the OODA categories.

- *When are they required on the journey?* This requires the availability of the patient and the actors from the *Who* question as well as the enabling technology. Coordination is required in some form of planning or scheduling processes.

- *Where will the journey take place?* What are the touchpoints at home, in transit, or in the practice or hospital? A small question but with a big impact on the ability to keep as active as possible and on the flip side of the coin, the impact on health provisioning outside specialized buildings, such as practices and hospitals.

- *Which enabling technology resources are required in this journey and are they available for use as intended?* The enabling technology consists of the traditional medical equipment, although now connected more and more to devices carried around by people, as we described in *Chapter 1, Understanding (the Need for) Transformation*, categorized as the **Internet of Things** (**IoT**). We are experiencing many innovations in the field of healthcare and it is these innovations that make the transformation possible. The *Which* question is key to enabling a great HeX with the platform.

- *How to make it work?* How are the workflows made with seamless interoperability and integrated interactions? The answers to this question are the customer objectives as input for the specifications. This also includes the objectives for the following:

  - User interfaces

  - Data availability and accessibility

  - Interactions for well-defined communication, coordination, control, and command

  - Connectivity between the resources

To recap, the first six questions starting with a *W* provide the specifications for the interactions. The *how* question translates these to fulfill the platform interaction given the resources, time, and place that we have defined.

Explaining the JIM

In this section, we will explain how to use the JIM, a method that emerged from the daily practice of the authors. It projects customer journeys on the seven *W*-questions, starting with the following figure:

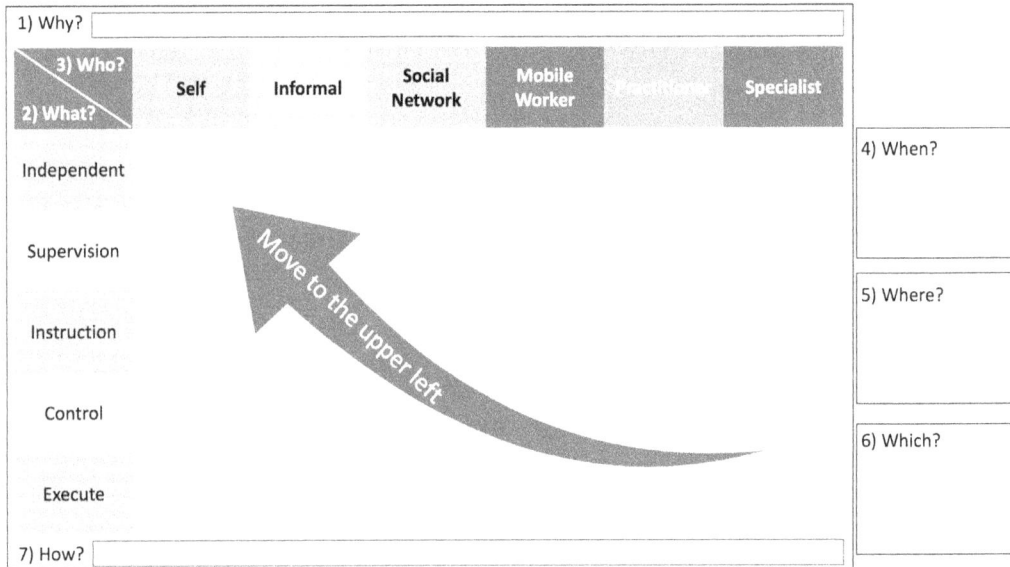

Figure 8.2 – JIM for plotting touchpoints on the health journey

The JIM starts with the question of *why* a health journey is needed, with a purpose such as rehabilitation from injury. With this purpose in mind, the touchpoints of the journey are plotted in the matrix with the two axes. On the horizontal axis are the interactions divided into *who* is doing the interaction, in terms of classes of skills and costs. It starts with the patient, followed by the informal caregiver, social network, remote or mobile workers, and practitioners, and ends with the medical specialists. This ordinal sequence in costs can be used to define a lean journey with action shifted to the left as much as possible.

The vertical axis represents the intensity of care needed to classify the types of *what* activities. It ranges from independent self-care via supervision of the patient's actions or instructing the patient step by step to controlling the actions of the patient hands-on or activities being executed by someone other than the patient. Supervision means just attending to see whether activities are done correctly and the expected results are obtained. Instructing means active communication with the patient. Control is, for example, safeguarding safety or physically helping the patient, and executing is about the patient taking a passive role and somebody else acting and taking care. Think of a nurse giving an injection. Obviously, lower intensity of care is better if possible, as this will have lower costs. The center of gravity of the journey must be moved to the upper left as much as possible given the circumstances. Notice that both axes are about someone and not something – in other words, they are about human activity and interactions. Human interactions are in the touchpoints of the journey.

Each matrix cell (the *Who* or *What* classifications) describes the OODA activity interaction at a touchpoint in the journey, with *When* and *Where* added, and with *Which* enabling technology. For example, in the **Mobile Worker/Supervision** matrix cell, we *Observe* whether the patient is taking their medication at home (*Where*) on time (*When*) by monitoring the alarm from the medication dispenser (the *Which* enabling technology). If required, in the case of medication not being taken (*Orient*), remember or instruct the patient to take the medication (implicit guidance to *Act*).

The interaction definition also mentions a device or thing, a medication dispenser (*Which*). These dispensers contain medicines that are required for each medication moment. For diseases such as Parkinson's, the exact timing of medication for the individual patient can increase the effectiveness significantly, resulting in being able to be more active. This kind of dispenser is usually placed at home (*Where*) and connected (*How*) via the internet to a pharmacy, for example. The *How* question is about the digital interaction, interoperability, and integration to enable the health journey to be a good experience.

Let's make this tangible in an example given in *Figure 8.3* of a complete journey where we have a patient that needs to recover from a knee operation:

- The target is that a patient is exercising as part of rehabilitation treatment after surgery. The aim is that the patient is doing these exercises at a time that is convenient. The patient can do the exercises at home with the use of a tablet to show them instructions. The exercises are recorded on video and it is requested that they fill in a questionnaire with the VAS score. The patient's aim is to walk again soon and be able to go to the supermarket.

- The observation is focusing on the pain experienced. If, for example, the exercises are done as part of recovery after an intervention such as surgery, then the exercises shouldn't jeopardize the healing of the wound. The VAS score and video taken of the exercise give a good indication of the amount of pain. It's the partner of the patient who is attending to the task of evaluating this and if required, sends a message to the practitioner.

- The practitioner receives the VAS score, video, and message from the partner and decides to decrease or increase the pain medication. This decision is processed via a workflow including the pharmacist and instructions are given to the partner, who attends to giving the medication manually.

This results in the following JIM. We recognize the OODA activities in *Figure 8.1*, but now in the context of the answers to the seven types of questions:

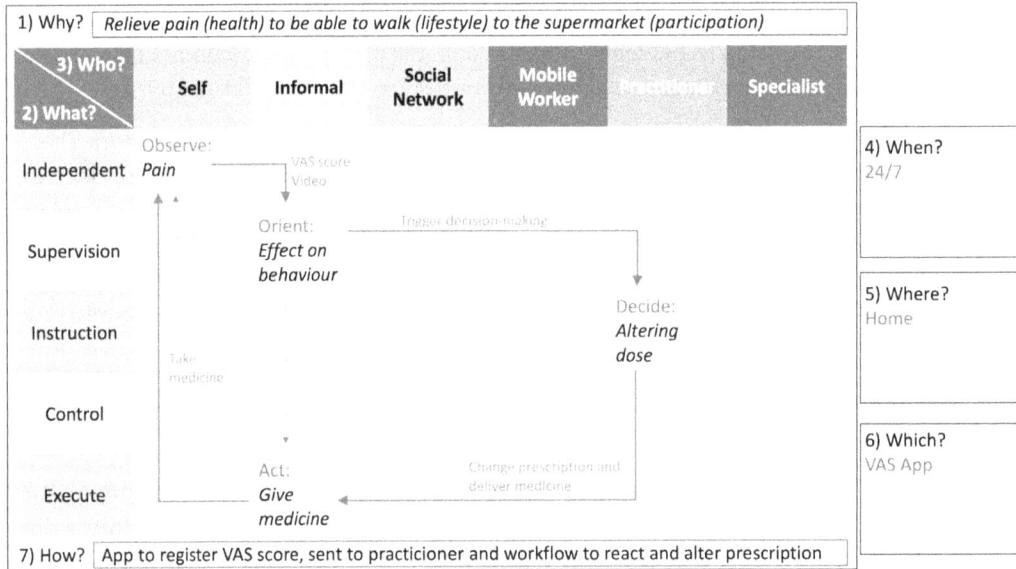

Figure 8.3 – A JIM with rehabilitation journey OODA loops

We learned in *Chapter 6, Applying the Panarchy Principle*, that resources have to be available so that people are not frustrated in the transformation process. The required enabling systems have to work.

Digital enablers determined in the JIM example given include the following:

- Tablet or smartphone with an exercise app including the VAS questionnaire and video app
- **Electronic Patient Registration (EPR)**
- Planner(s) of the closed-loop medication process
- Connectivity

By defining the journey using interactions at the touchpoints in terms of OODA loops, an integrated view is created of patient-centric care provisioning. This integrated view is used to design the architecture for the development of interoperability-enabling digital technology. We will explore this further in the following sections.

Enabling the journey with DevOps

In the previous section, we described how to define a journey that a patient could go through to be able to participate fully in society again, delivered by the ecosystem of networked care. For this, we need DevOps, in that technology is dynamically and carefully allocated to the specific journey in the ecosystem and made available, easy to use, and fully managed so that users needn't worry about the appropriate support of devices and software.

We need a process to steer the DevOps process for this purpose. Maybe in one organization that is in place, however, the DevOps process and the demands of the complete ecosystem are different. Sometimes referred to as the whole system in the room, with all organizations involved we have indeed caught the complete story of the ecosystem.

The mechanism is the 4Care part of DevOps4Care, Support, Experience, Value and Tell as in *Figure 3.3*. The feedback loop consists of the following:

- Support by managing the availability and use of the deployed, enabling technology

- Experience by observing how interactions in tasks and activities occur in practice

- Value by evaluating the experience compared to what is expected and required

- Tell by communicating with users about how valuable the outcomes of DevOps are and how these outcomes can be improved

Let's elaborate on this a bit further, as it is essential in DevOps4Care in networked care.

Support: Normally, for each care provider after deployment, including the onboarding of end users, the operation consists of organizing support with a proper service desk, including the self-help portal, **Frequently Asked Questions (FAQs)**, and chat functions, but also the involvement of the digicoach role in the extended support team. When collaborating in the ecosystem and ensuring closed OODA loops, this becomes more complicated. The challenge is to coordinate all operations as if they were done under one entity. In *Chapter 9, Working with Complex (System of) Systems*, we will come back to this.

Experience: The experience is determined by the use of all enablers such as the tablet, app, and connectivity used in the interactions during the journeys that we described. Experience is measured by how effectively the enablers can be used to realize the cross-organization OODA loops. Besides the objective fulfillment of a process, it is important to know whether something is not working or experienced well. We should not solely address the technical side but also look for what might be the underlying cause with the Knoster, Rogers, Moore, and Mezirow models in mind and address the problem, need, or inhibition point for a solution, as described in *Chapter 6, Applying the Panarchy Principle.*

Value: Next is the value of the experience in terms of the value creation stages given in *Chapter 3, Unfolding the Complexity of Transformation*:

- Personal value – as in, job satisfaction and security
- Fulfilling the requirements and ability to support the team
- Supporting the activities in the workflows within the guidelines and protocols
- Determining the results of treatment or intervention
- Customer satisfaction in terms of the quality of care delivered
- Improving the quality of life of the patient
- Outlook on the participation of the patient

For each of these stages, instruments are available to capture the value. The **Groninger Wellbeing Indicator (GWI)** (by Joris Slaets), consisting of two questions, is a good example of such an instrument:

- Which of these areas are important to you?

  - Good sleep and rest
  - Enjoying eating and drinking
  - Pleasant relationships and contacts
  - Being active
  - Caring for yourself
  - Being yourself
  - Feeling healthy in body and mind
  - Enjoyable living

- Are you satisfied in these areas?

  It's an example of a true HeX used by some nursing homes in the Netherlands. To close the feedback loop, the third question is, *if not satisfied, what are we going to do about it?*

For example, a person is hiding possessions such as hearing aid, glasses, and dentures before going to sleep because they are important for eating and having contact. In the morning, the patient forgets where they were hidden, due to a memory-related condition. It leads to the wrong conclusion that they have been stolen, causing anxiety. Nursing personnel can't always find these possessions either, taking up valuable nursing time either way.

The solution was to *hide* the possessions in a secure locker for this person before sleeping and return them in the morning. In this case, it was the interaction with the next of kin using the GWI that gathered that the patient suffered from anxiety. Together with next of kin, the care staff oriented on why this was happening, explored possible solutions, and decided to act. This was registered in the **electronic record** (**EHR**) to be used in the daily planning of nursing activities. In this case, it resulted in a happier patient and less burden on the nursing staff for the final 2 years of this elderly person's life. Fewer care activities meant an improved quality of life in this case!

> Tip
>
> For a deeper understanding of the Dutch healthcare system and its challenges in terms of digital transformation, read *The transformation of elderly care: The impact of digitalization* by Harry Woldendorp. It can be found here: `https://www.google.co.in/books/edition/The_transformation_of_elderly_care/91czEAAAQBAJ?hl=en`.

Tell: The final step of feedback in DevOps is communicating what can be improved. This is the game-changing mechanism driving the transformation that we know so well from DevOps and agile working, again, in concert with the entire ecosystem. Here, community builders have a big task – organizing so that everyone involved in a closed OODA loop is heard. A JIM session is designed to do that. It will give a common understanding of the requirements needed to design and develop the enabling platform as a whole.

The feedback will drive the development of the microservices. Ultimately, somewhere in the future, the digicoach, e-nurse, or lead user can detect what improvements are wanted by zero-coding the microservices themselves. This requires building a digital twin following the shared mental models first. This will also take several steps to achieve. The people, teams, and organizations will have to learn the skills and go through their own transformational learning process.

At this point, we will refer once again to the **Customer Objectives, Application, Functional, Conceptual, Realization through Reasoning Exploring Qualifying Specifying** (**CAFCR REQS**) model. Exploration is the layer where the stories are told and a priori solutions are suggested. Creating explicit exploration JIM sessions within the organization and collaborating is a good start to implementing the communication link between care and DevOps. These sessions can evolve by using simulations with the digital shadow to determine the impact of possible solutions and prepare to code the improvements in the next release, following the trend of automated DevOps.

The results of the JIM sessions are the input for development where, once again, developers from all transitions have to coordinate the actions and pace. Testing will have to be done not only on their own component or system but will also have to be fully integrated to enable the closed OODA loop:

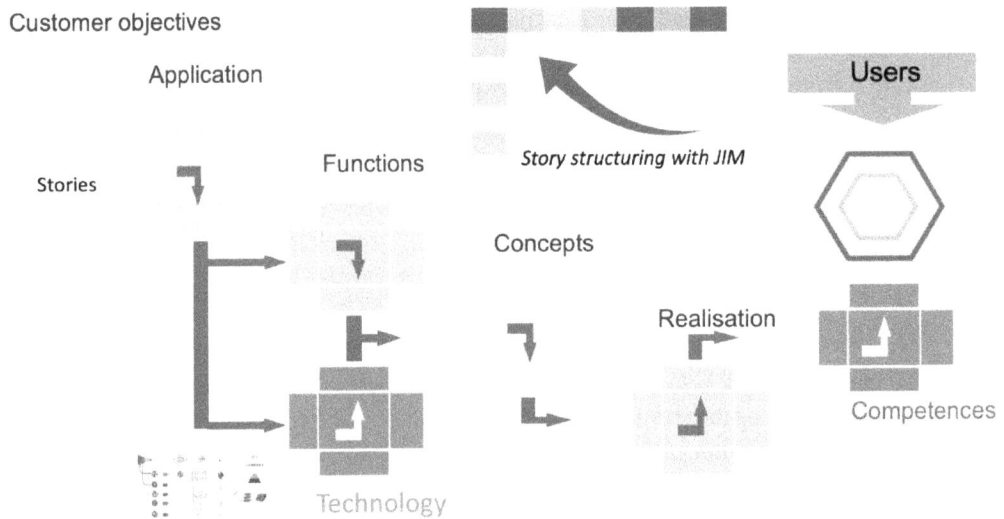

Figure 8.4 – JIM stories as the input requirement for platform development

Here, the systems engineers come in again, especially in engineering management, which focuses on how to design, integrate, and manage complex systems over their life cycles.

A coalition of organizations grows from an ad hoc group via collaboration towards cooperation with ever more complex systems. It will take time to learn how to manage these complex systems together.

In the end, it should result in daily or even hourly releases to follow the dynamics required for adapting and forming care networks based on a person's health experience. We will come back to this in the coming chapters.

In this section, we discussed the different interactions and actors in the OODA activities to realize the 4Care feedback to DevOps. These actors all fulfill particular roles that must be defined in the systems that we will be using. Actors with different roles as patients or as part of the TEC teams – together with the responsibility to provide the closed OODA loops. The following section will explain how to define these roles and why this is important.

Exploring the roles of team members and patients

Now, why is it important to define roles from the perspective of OODA? We already saw that we have various actors defining actions based on observations and orientations, leading to decisions. These actors can perform optimally when they have access to the right tools and data. Care is optimized when actors work together in the chain or network of care, using the right tools and data, as it is integrated into that chain. The interactions in the activities in the chain define the care and the execution of the activities by the right actors defines the quality of the care. Actors and activities need to be able to interact.

Roles need classification in order to be assigned the right attributes, to be identified properly, and to get access to the right resources in terms of the closed OODA loops along the journey.

We therefore use a known way of working in healthcare in which the OODA loop is intrinsically present – social alarming. Social alarming is well established and therefore a good model for getting a shared understanding of redefining the roles. It provides the structure to build the OODA loop, as social alarming contains all steps required.

The responsibilities of the service chain process from onboarding, providing a service, to ending the service with social alarming or TEC mechanisms in general are well defined in standards such as the European CEN/TC 431. There is a firm focus on the users ensuring an improved level of health experience in the health journey.

The standard CEN/TC 431 achieves this by working with all interconnected parts in the entire service chain, or loop as we call it for social care alarms. A link to this standard is provided in the *Further reading* section.

Technology and organization structure independence are important features of this standard – the service model for social care alarms. Using this service model, we – instead of reading social alarming and reacting to alarms – can interpret it as health service reacting to events.

The technology-enabled health service typically follows this path:

- Initiated, resulting in acquiring the required enabling technology to enable the defined loops of the initiated journey
- Used in the journey of healthcare provisioning enabled by management and support
- It is assessed whether to continue, change, abort, or re-initialize the healthcare service
- Ended, resulting in the healthcare service being terminated

For our purposes, it suffices to distinguish the enabling roles:

- Supplier of equipment, devices, and application services
- Installation and activation service of endpoint equipment used at the premises of the actors

- Health event monitor and action dispatcher in the care network, such as present-day remote **Intensive Care Units** (**ICUs**), ambulance response, and other community alarm or telecare services.

- Technical **Operations** (**Ops**) coordinator of the end-to-end management of the feedback loops

- Provider of the technology-enabled response health services

Each of these plays its role in the deployment of services, including onboarding, supporting, and managing the enabling technologies. With the enabling technology in place, the user or actor roles in provisioning the actual journey with health services are divided into the following:

- Observe whether an event has occurred defined in the journey

- Orient what this event signifies

- Decide on who is going to respond and how

- Act accordingly as defined in the journey

Here, the OODA shared mental model comes in on the technology side too. To assure the proper working of the enabling technology for the closed OODA loop healthcare provisioning, the same sequence is used:

- Observe whether an incident has occurred, disturbing the proper working of the enabling technology in such a way that the feedback loops are going to be affected

- Orient on what the root cause of the incident is

- Decide on who is going to respond and restore the proper functioning of the enabling technology

- Act accordingly to restore the feedback loop

In this way, the processes mirror each other on both the medical and technical side, creating a better mutual understanding.

Of course, this has to be managed end to end over the entire platform.

Summary

In this chapter, we focused on the members of the different TEC teams and their interactions. We explored the roles and tasks of these teams and how they can support the patient during the health journey. These teams operate in ecosystems – hence, they need to be interoperable and interact with different actors in the entire health journey that provides the health experience for the patient. The teams are supported by technology, so we must ensure that operations are in place to assist the teams in working with technology and help whenever an issue occurs. Lastly, the technology needs to be improved per evolving demands and the requirements of the patient. This is exactly what DevOps4Care envisions.

In this chapter, we introduced the JIM. By answering the questions *why*, *when*, *where*, and *which*, the right care is defined. Obviously, this is done by observing the patient and orienting the situation or circumstances, the steps we discussed in the OODA loop.

We discussed how to capture the stories from the users as input for the development process, spanning the whole ecosystem, and we discussed how roles are divided in both the healthcare provisioning and enabling technology operations in this kind of ecosystem.

We will discuss interoperability and interaction in those ecosystems further in the next chapter by deep-diving into the concept of micro-enterprises and their enabling platforms.

Further reading

- *Multi-Cloud Architecture and Governance* by Jeroen Mulder, Packt Publishing

- *Big Data for Architects* by Bhavuk Chawla, Packt Publishing, 2021

- *IoT and Edge Computing for Architects* by Perry Lea, Packt Publishing, 2020

- *CEN/TC 431 - SERVICE CHAIN FOR SOCIAL CARE ALARMS*, CEN: `https://standards.iteh.ai/catalog/tc/cen/732920f7-04dc-4e4c-b100-788999bc1bce/cen-tc-431`

- We recommend reading the work of Maaike Kleinsmann on this topic of common understanding: `https://www.tudelft.nl/io/over-io/personen/kleinsmann-ms`

9
Working with Complex (System of) Systems

After our first job, it's time to consider our career. MoM TiSH is confident that we are ready to climb the corporate ladder.

We introduced the **Journey Interaction Matrix** (**JIM**) in *Chapter 8, Learning How Interaction Works in Technology-Enabled Care Teams*, to utilize OODA, which was introduced in *Chapter 7, Creating New Platforms with OODA*. Together, they provide a way to tell structured stories about the relationships between the activities in health journeys, executed by providers and the enablers. In this chapter, we will learn how to create a common understanding to integrate and transform into the top tread of TiSH, personal directed healthcare with the best-fitting solutions and systems, tread by tread.

The TiSH staircase and DevOps4Care enable users to tell compelling and understandable stories along the presented models. This allows developers to understand the needs to design each tread and build the enabling systems. We will address the integration and interoperability of these systems in the enabling platform, the two critical issues to solve in any complex ecosystem. That requires understanding the technology, as well as the interaction of multi-disciplinary teams that work together from a care perspective. It's all part of TiSH and DevOps4Care.

In this chapter, we're going to cover the following main topics:

- Building the **Technology-Enabled Care** (**TEC**) teams
- Introducing integration in networked care teams of teams
- Cross-walking integration and interoperability relations
- Applying SSP, governance, and operations
- Integrating TEC teams with patient-centric networks

Building the Technology-Enabled Care (TEC) teams

With the JIM at our disposal, we can define the interactions between teams in terms of OODA activities. In the following figure, we added the JIM to the third tread of TiSH. This enables a care organization to define the care processes in OODA activities and have the required capacity within each team to provide the requested care to patients. Given this capacity, the teams have to be integrated into the activities of other teams when involved in networked care.

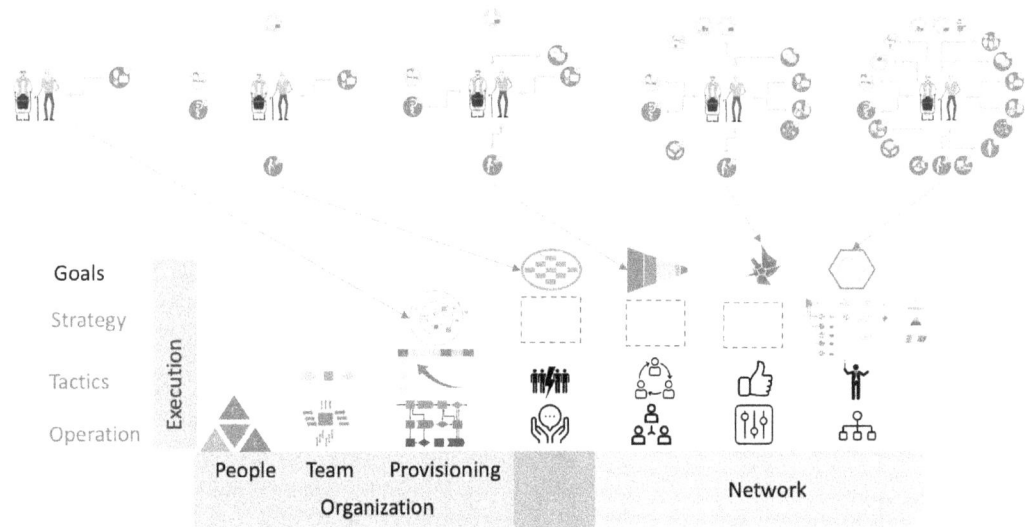

Figure 9.1 – Interactions between TEC teams and their (OODA) activities

We are not going to describe the professional medical or social procedures, but rather a strategy for the generic functionality and characteristics of how to integrate the different care teams in the following types of care networks we defined previously:

- In ad hoc networks, case management needs to know what the other care providers are doing. The actions of other care providers are observed to see what they do as part of their own OODA loop. They communicate to each other about what they do or have done.

- In stepped care, several teams make joint decisions on the health OODA loop, requiring coordination and collaboration between the care teams.

- In integrated care, social and medical care teams are integrated. The teams manage the lifestyle OODA loop, enhanced with diagnostics and orient on what the best actions for the lifestyle of a particular patient are.

- In directed care, all care teams' treatments or other interventions are commanded from the jointly observed participation OODA loop.

To visualize the nested OODA loops for integrating the different teams, the following diagram shows the hierarchy of the OODA loops, each related to the type of networked care:

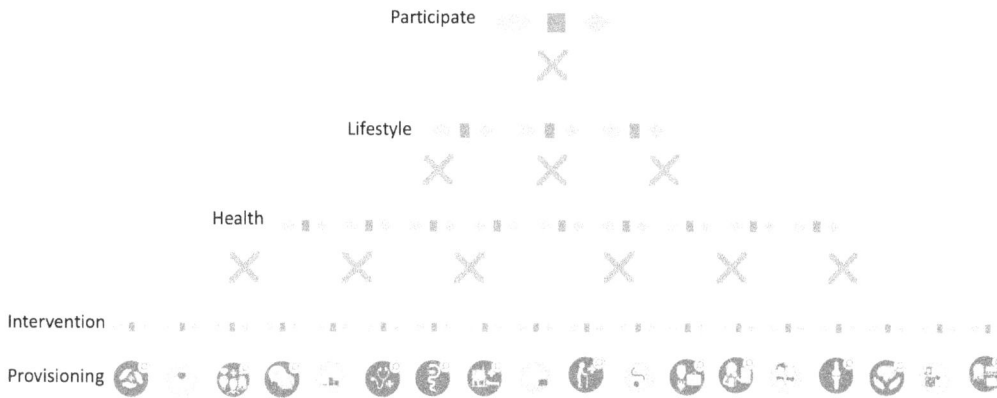

Figure 9.2 – OODA loop hierarchy

In the final chapter of this book, we will do an exercise on nested OODA loops as the main design for networked care.

Now that we have decomposed the TEC team into the components of roles and OODA activities using the JIM, it's time to compose the TEC teams and the networked care. First, remember what we discussed in *Chapter 6, Applying the Panarchy Principle,* regarding Tuckman's views on how the team is built with forming, storming, norming, performing, and adjourning steps, and must be able to express their care processes in terms of OODA activities. These activities must be mirrored in the technology.

Next, this team must be digitally skilled. These teams need to become digital centaurs in the care networks, which will take time. TEC teams operate in networks, using platform services that they can dynamically scale around the patients using technology.

The next section will address this.

Introducing integration in networked care teams of teams

It's time to talk about micro-enterprises and **3EO**, the **Entrepreneurial Ecosystem Enabling Organization**. We already briefly mentioned Rendanheyi as an agile way to unbundle and rebundle organizations to suit the patient's needs, realized in the Moments of Truth on the health journey's touchpoints. The question is how?

For each network tread, we will provide an example. The first is case management, which is shown in the following diagram:

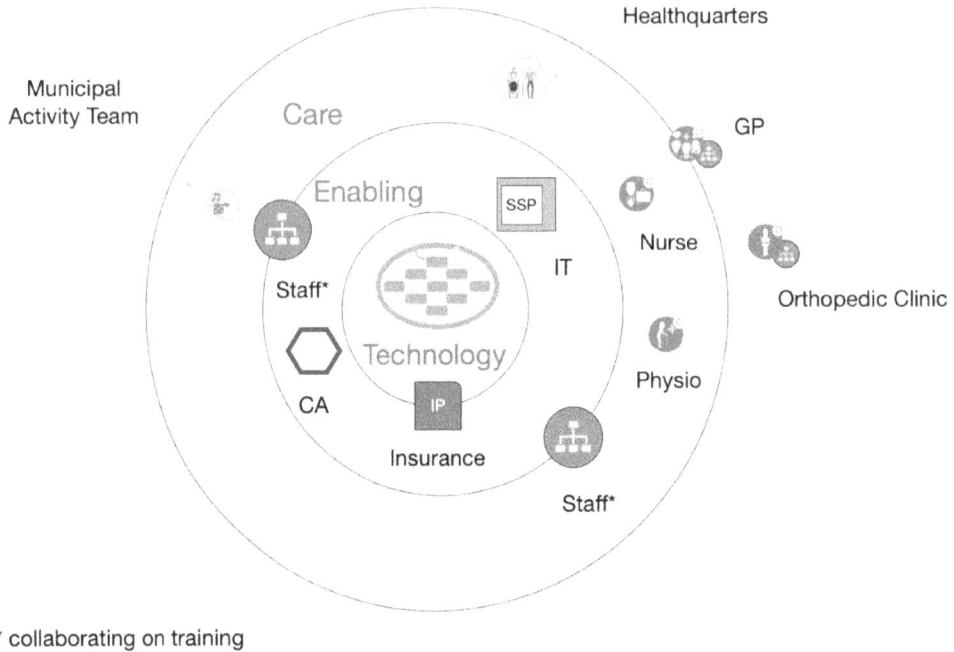

* collaborating on training

Figure 9.3 – Teams in case management

Figure 9.3 shows a playing field with **Technology** in the inner circle, **Enabling** entities in the middle circle, and **Care** providers in the outer circle. Other teams or organizations can be outside these circles.

The patient has its healthquarters – analogous to headquarters – at home. Together with the partner, they are their own case manager (self-management) to arrange the care they need. In this example, we have a patient who is recovering after an intervention replacing a hip. The intervention is done in the orthopedic clinic, but the rehabilitation is done at home.

The patient and their partner have a subscription paid by the insurance company to arrange the care they need. The subscription is issued by an enabling organization, a rehabilitation center. The subscription covers a nursing team and physiotherapists, working together with the **General Practitioner** (**GP**).

The binding party here is the healthcare insurance company. They provide the governance for the **Integration Platform** (**IP**). Through their purchasing power, they can specify what capabilities and functionalities of communication are required for proper case management. Obviously, all parties must be compliant with the guardrails that have been laid out in governmental regulations.

To make sure that the communication requirements are met, an independent **Certifying Agency (CA)** certifies all players within their circles of influence.

The rehabilitation center has also made arrangements with the municipality, which has a specific team organizing activities such as cycling, walking, and playing games. Both the rehabilitation center and the municipality have decided to work together on training their personnel but have their own department for **Human Resources Management (HRM)**.

By just looking at the department and team level of organizations, we have already digitally unbundled the organizations. This will help with the organizational unbundling when this is required.

If we go one step further to stepped care, the playing field changes. It's shown in the following diagram:

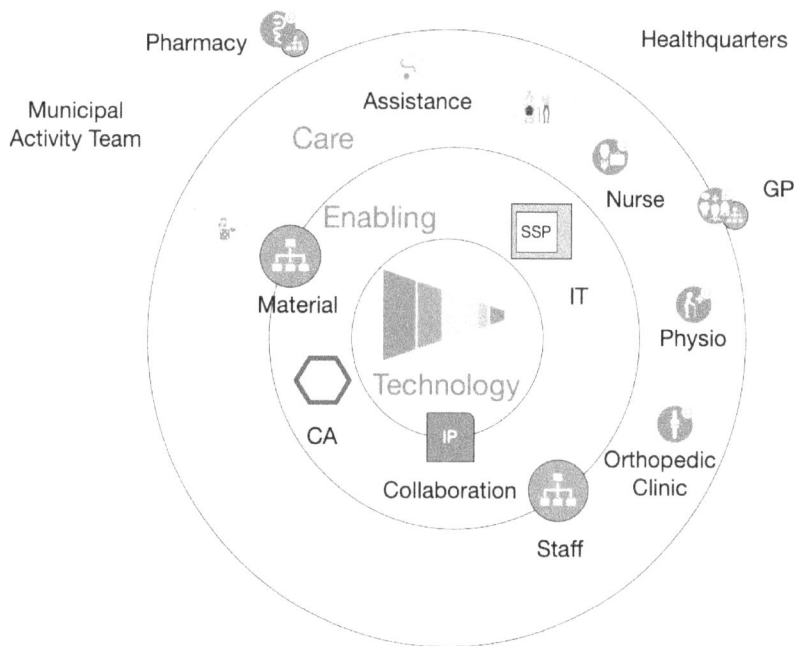

Figure 9.4 – Teams in stepped care

Like the Danish Naerkliniken that we already introduced in the first chapters of this book, a formal collaboration is established between the municipality, the clinic, practices in the neighborhood, and the rehabilitation center. The GP is involved and the pharmacy acts as an external supplier.

In the collaboration, it was decided that enabling staff has to be trained jointly. The clinic and rehab center provide the human resources related to the collaboration and the municipality provides all materials for use at home. The assistance for housekeeping from the municipality is also part of the collaboration.

In the collaboration, they use the guiding hand of the insurance company for governance. The use of CAs to certify all entities using the **Shared Services Platform (SSP)** is retained.

Next, we evolve to integrated care, represented in the following diagram:

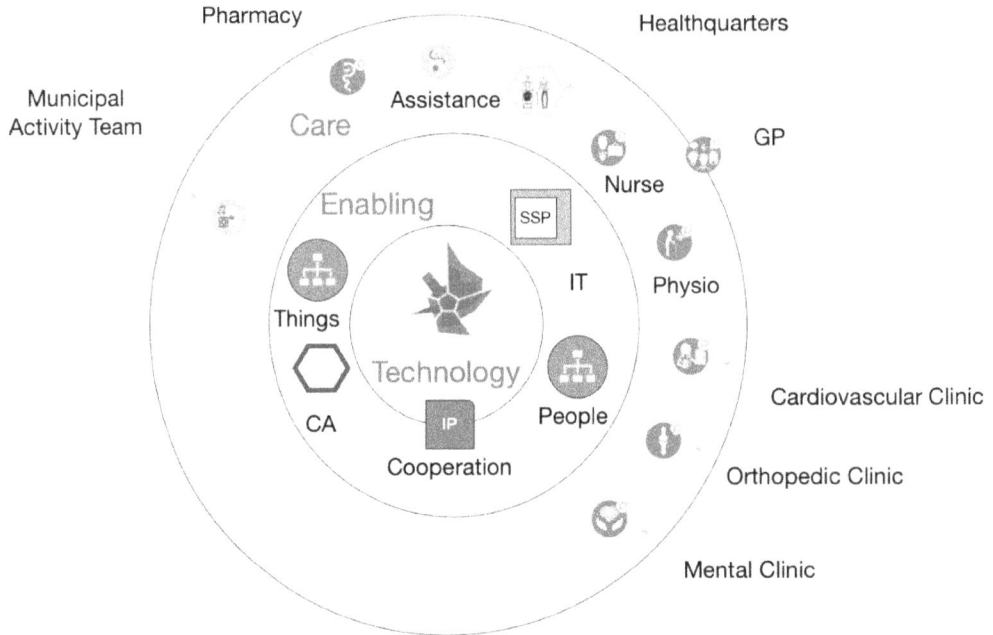

Figure 9.5 – Teams in integrated care

If we want to go into integrated care, then more disciplines must be involved to cooperate. This time, a cooperation is founded that will be responsible for all platforms to support the entities. One example of cooperation is that all equipment or things required for use at home can be ordered by any team from the online platform.

The same applies to human resources with a platform to assign tasks to individuals across the teams. The Roamler Care platform that we discussed in *Chapter 8, Learning How Interaction Works in Technology-Enabled Care Teams*, provides this. The HRM department is absorbed in the teams, like with the Buurtzorg concept.

Last but not least (in fact, delivering the most value for the patient) is directed care, which is shown in the following diagram:

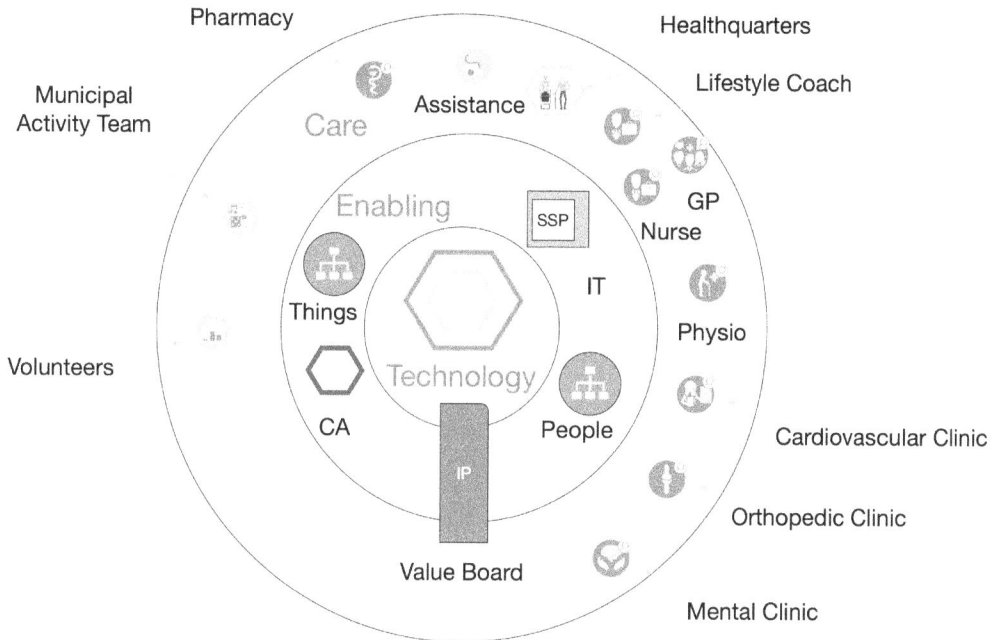

Figure 9.6 – Teams in directed care

In directed care, the healthquarters of anyone can direct the care resources via the SSP. This can be highly autonomous as health trackers predict when some form of care is required.

The IP is now governed by a value board responsible for the population management of the region. All teams are in fact free to independently develop to serve the population as best as possible. The Amazon Care approach has a lot of these characteristics, the population being the workforce of Amazon itself.

Integrating TEC teams with patient-centric networks

Integrating the TEC teams means interaction between the OODA activities, at least the internal activities and especially the OODA activities in networked care. We need nurses, therapists, practitioners, and doctors in the teams to be interoperable. We also need to enable supporting staff to manage the services to create the **Health eXperience (HeX)** journeys.

Although this integration is on the medical side, it must also be realized on the enabling technical side. To be able to build understanding on both sides, we present an overview of the entities on both sides in the following figure:

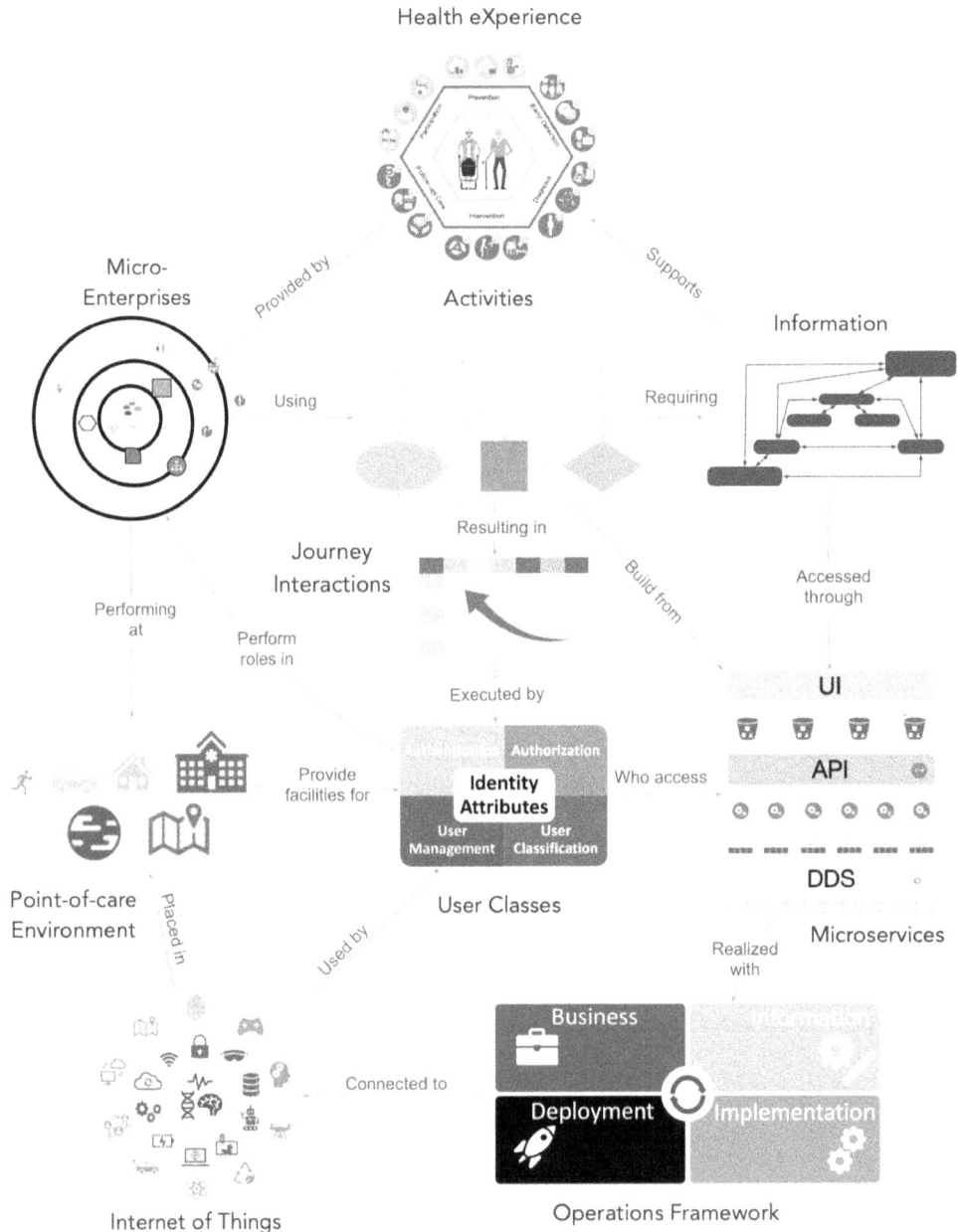

Figure 9.7 – Entity relation diagram for journeys, providers, and the enablers

To be able to translate the integration and interoperability into enabling services of the platform, we need to recognize the care provisioning entities in the upper part and the enabling entities in the lower part. The awareness of these entities helps with understanding the stories we tell each other. The transformation task force will have to organize common understanding sessions to build a shared mental model for the DevOps4Care process. We use the **Entity Relations Diagram** (**ERD**) for this purpose. The entities are divided into 4Care entities and Ops entities. Together, they will be developed.

On the care provisioning (4Care) business side, we identify the following:

- The HeX on treatment, health, lifestyle, and participation.

- Information represented by the **International Classification of Functioning, Disability**, **and Health (ICF)** model and the medical information elements it contains, including other types of information, such as for scheduling, payment, quality, and logistics. For example, medical data entities, datasets, and their granularity are defined in **Clinical Information Models (CIMs)**.

- Activities from the OODA loops consisting of protocols and guidelines translated into workflows of tasks using defined processes based on, for example, the insights of the **Interoperable Health Enterprise (IHE)**.

- Micro-enterprises consisting of TEC teams and the enabling teams, such as for HRM and IT.

- Journey interactions of people as patients or people who want to improve their health, lifestyle, and participation in the touchpoints as part of the care activities.

The enabling entities are as follows:

- **Point-of-care environments**: Care is indeed traditionally provided in hospitals or on the premises of the caregivers. House calls can be made by GPs and ambulant nurses, but only for a limited set of care activities. But care is increasingly provided anywhere on the globe as things such as wearables and implants become much more common. The environments of the Point-of-care are therefore becoming ever more challenging.

- **Internet of Things technology**: The Internet of Things, which we talked about in *Chapter 2, Exploring Relevant Technologies for Healthcare*, is not merely things connected to the internet. It often combines all sorts of technology, such as in a technology warehouse, into very sophisticated and capable devices. It ranges from a common smartwatch to an artificial pancreas, as well as home dialysis or breathing equipment, CT or MRI scanners in hospitals, and DNA sequencers in the lab. It is here where breakthrough innovations are taking place. For instance, smart pills already exist that send back information about where they are in the body, or defibrillator delivery drones give a rapid response. This will shift healthcare increasingly outside the traditional buildings.

- **User classes**: User classes refer to which types of users are involved in the journey. They have to be classified into distinctive classes, people who are the receivers of care, next of kin, volunteers, community workers, care professionals of all sorts, and supporting staff. Not only people but also increasingly devices and their algorithms are classes on their own. These devices work increasingly autonomously. A simple example is a chatbot.

These classes are managed as users of resources to enable the care teams. For this, users must identify themselves with the right attributes to be authenticated. Once authenticated, authorization to access the resources can be granted.

- **Microservices**: Microservices are the backbone of digitization and interoperability. The modular setup consists of the systems of engagement with the **User Interface** (**UI**) and the systems of record as a **Distributed Data System** (**DDS**), distributed in several domains – hospital, personal, private, and public, to name the most common. The systems of engagement, systems of intelligence, and systems of record are connected with **Application Programming Interfaces** (**APIs**). This separates data from the application to provide better security and flexibility to reuse data and create data flows along the journey and use the data in research.

- **Operations framework**: An operations framework is used to define the complete processes, roles, procedures, tools, and activities to govern, design, deploy, train, manage, and continuously improve all IT services. It's a guide to a network's governance and assurance of operations on concepts, principles, UI/UX, API, AI algorithms, data, security, and connectivity. The framework sets out the way the network enables care by forming the back office for the microservices, user classes, and connected Internet of Things placed in the Point of Care Environments. For the best healthcare provisioning, an excellent operational framework is needed to ensure collaboration with best-of-class IT services to motivate and enable all involved people. It's the Ops in DevOps.

The ERD shown in *Figure 9.7* shows the relations of the platform between the entities.

This ERD (from TAFIM, the precursor to TOGAF) is used as the foundation for architecture preferably set up from the start to be able to evolve the patient-centric network into the desired SSP.

We use the OODA loops to organize the teams around the patient; how do we mirror that in the IT resources of the platform? What technological topics are important to be aware of as the transformation task force? Let's dive into it.

IT resources

The IT resources need to be one step ahead of the most advanced organization in the network. But here, we have to say that this is rarely the case. Here, the need for a common vision of the future based on a common understanding becomes apparent. We will address this in the next chapter. The consequence is that the topology of the IT infrastructure must be futureproof in terms of the transformation treads ahead. A multi-cloud strategy is therefore a must as the SSP will evolve from micro-enterprises originating from different, more traditional organizations, each having its own choice of cloud. These can be public clouds such as Azure and AWS, but also private stacks hosted in privately owned data centers or hosting providers. The first step to take is to prepare the modular microservices for interoperability between the environments in these clouds, but also all subsequent integration levels have to be prepared for.

Integration levels are defined on the business side by the OODA loops and the accompanying level of Systems of Systems for the technology on the other side. It's this combination that has to be addressed in the common understanding.

One field of knowledge for this is decision support systems.

> **Tip**
>
> Read the publication on decision support, *Decision Support Systems and Management Information System*, by Pawan Thakur and Ram Kumar.

Trust

Another topic for common understanding is trust. Every organization should build trust in the users by having excellent privacy, security, and UX. All actors in the HeXagon have to communicate with each other in a secure way.

That starts with each organization having its own trust domain. So, how do we unbundle this? By having each entity operating from its own domain with zero trust between the domains. For each person or device, it is possible to get access to the required microservices via the API, including the preferred **Operating Systems (OSs)** and UI.

With the creation of trusted domains, we're moving from one domain to confined personal domains. The step toward unbundling becomes easy. The organization becomes just another attribute of an identity. With this, we are already getting close to the next version of the internet, called **Web3**, using blockchain technology to decentralize the web. It could be used to grant every identity its own personal domain, shielded as a block and providing a greater level of security and privacy. But the benefits are there: patients owning their own domain and granting access to actors in the care network on demand.

We are creating a patient's health data space domain. In the HeXagon, a practitioner logs into that patient's domain, where they have permission to look for other data to be used in the therapy or other type of intervention. This is the opposite of a patient logging into all different care providers. Prepare to flip the domain inside out. The consequence of this is that every active entity has to be aware of what they are doing – it's *they* since we're talking about both humans and devices – and what data is being stored.

If actors can be anywhere, so can data. We won't have monolithic data stores anymore, but distributed data. The next challenge is how to find the right data when it's distributed. You can use an index to find where your data is or search all databases on related data. The index method is quicker and can be recorded with each event between actors. Searching will also include derived or processed data. So, both ways are probably needed for access to complete data.

For example, algorithm micro-AI services will need the required data and will search for it. Technologies such as DDS used in other sectors such as aerospace become relevant for healthcare too.

The way it works is that an actor logs into the required domains, getting access to conditions such as authorization and circumstances such as legal relationship. An actor can publish information and/or subscribe to information required for the task at hand.

From the start, it is best to give this ultimate perspective attention and create the design space for the end goal. Also, unbundle staff organizations in the IT domain to prepare for the coming rebundling around the patient's needs.

This includes the IT department preparing to support the emerging SSP. The IT department can take the lead on the transformation by first collaborating and then forming a cooperation to ultimately support the individual patient by setting up the support on rigorous **Identity and Access Management (IAM)** and digital services.

Identity management

The next main topic is how to get access to the data. Every person or thing that needs data for their activity needs to find and get cleared for access in line with their roles in the activity. The main dilemma is, on the one hand, protecting data, and on the other hand, providing access to those who need it. In our practice, we see care providers struggling to give access to personnel outside their own organization. What we need is identity management across all care providers, across the silos.

Before we dive into the specific roles of professionals and patients, we must define what roles are. In IT, roles are associated with identities. But to make it a bit more complex: identities are not just people. Anything can be an identity. In the previous chapter, we discussed how to disentangle or unbundle healthcare services into microservices, allowing the patient to acquire the right service at the desired time. This way, we can dynamically scale resources to provide care.

A microservice is a resource, but it doesn't run on itself. It needs infrastructure and software. It may need a device and it will certainly need network connectivity. Lastly, it needs a user to drive the service and a receiver that benefits from the service. All of these are identities, and they fulfill a role.

This concept might be a bit hard to understand if you aren't an IT expert, so we'll try to make it more specific.

Both the care provider, for instance, a nurse, and the patient are identities. To use care services, they will need access to these services. They might need access to an app on a tablet or a mobile phone. But we only need to grant access to data that is relevant to this specific nurse and patient. Hence, we need to specify who they are, what their role is, and what this role requires. We might even want to be specific about when they need data or where and on what kind of device they are allowed to view data.

A lot of smartphones already have an app that shows relevant health data. That app might collect data from a smartwatch, but it can also hold the data that is entered by a GP or a pharmacy. The patient has access to that app and that data, but also the GP. However, the GP might not be allowed to view data that originated from the smartwatch.

This is where IAM comes in. In our example, we have several identities: patient, provider, GP, pharmacist, and the smartwatch or the tablet and the app itself that needs access to data. Who and what is allowed to view data, based on what role? When and where is access allowed, based on what conditions? This is only about the access, but we need an extra step: we must authenticate the identities – make sure that the identity is whoever or whatever they or it claim(s) to be.

This must be very fine-grained since we are organizing the healthcare to be dynamically scalable into micro-enterprises, changing networks and ecosystems, and microservices. All of this requires management with those end-to-end managed services. We don't want the nurse or the patient to be bothered by things such as IAM and authentication; it simply must be arranged. We need services that take care of the entire process: from login up to the presentation of the requested data. We need services that manage the functioning of the app, the security of the databases, and the establishment of network connectivity.

One important aspect of granting access to identities with specific roles is trust. If we grant access to identities, we have to first authenticate the role they have, verify that the identity is whoever they claim to be, and trust that they have the appropriate access. Identities should only have access to data that they are eligible to see and use. This is important for a lot of reasons: compliance with laws and regulations to start with. In IT, we use the zero-trust model and use micro-segmentation to enforce proper access, authorization, and authentication.

The most important principle in zero trust is **never trust, always verify**. In IT, this is typically translated into an architecture that authorizes and authenticates an identity by default. A zero-trust architecture has a single source of user identities. Users and devices are authenticated against that source, including the context, such as compliance with policies and the state of devices. Policies include rules to access an application and data within that application.

An extra line of defense is micro-segmentation, allowing architects to logically divide segments where applications and data reside. This prevents identities – users and devices – from simply hopping from one segment in a network to another without strong authorization and authentication. The identities and roles provided grant the proper access, after verification. These should be common rules in defining roles and access policies in healthcare.

Enabling integration in operations framework

Nothing will happen in the health journey if there are no operations in the background enabling healthcare with technology. We already introduced our TEC teams. This is a term that is also used by CENELEC, the European standardization body, in the framework for *service design and management and the development of management standards and shared values within and between the organizations engaged in the social alarm service chain.*

CENELEC uses TECOM derived from eTOM from TM Forum. The entity in *Figure 9.7* is a representation of their **Open Digital Architecture (ODA)**, which can be explored in detail online at `http://www.casewise.tmforum.org/evolve/statics/tmfmodel/index.html`.

It's a comprehensive operations framework including governance of, for instance, APIs used in the microservices. Again, for a common understanding, it suffices that the key principles are understood. So, what should this service look like? It's these enabling operations that provide the support services so that care workers can concentrate on the health journey and not have to worry about the technology that is used. Technology is water from a tap; it needs to be there, and it needs to work. However, to make that happen, the operations on all supporting entities and the logistics must be executed in an orchestrated way, allowing care workers to execute sense and response in events during the health journey. In fact, we can apply OODA here too: observe whether services are working for the users, orient on the detected service disturbances and user stories, decide on what measures to take, and act upon them. The users will recognize this approach. As operations become more complex with each tread, we also foresee a development in the operations framework, such as starting with TECOM, evolving to eTOM, using Ops4Care where user stories are readily understood by Ops, and using DevOps4Care when automated DevOps is added where users can no-code their services.

This concludes the dive into the technology. It's clear that it requires the skills of systems engineering and community building alike. In the next chapter, we will address this further by cross-walking the resulting integration and interoperability.

Cross-walking integration and interoperability relations

In *Chapter 3, Unfolding the Complexity of Transformation*, we first mentioned the terms interoperability and integration. Remember *Figure 3.5 – Structuring governance in healthcare systems*. Interoperability matters a lot to us. It's even the foundation for the transformation. Think of it as the HeX being created around touchpoints and interaction in each journey, this implicitly means that interoperability enables these interactions. The interoperability we are talking about is that between the OODA activities. These activities are overarching organizations and teams.

Using the ERD of *Figure 9.7*, we can describe the enabling entities step by step from components via systems to System of Systems and explore two essential topics: the interoperability and data domains and enabling integration along the ERD relations.

Understanding interoperability in data domains

Infrastructure must be interoperable from day one. This is the foundation. Systems need to be able to communicate with each other. Technologically, it means that systems must share protocols and interactive connections. But just interoperability of infrastructure doesn't mean by default that systems can communicate. They need to understand each other and understand each other's language. In terms of data, it means that we first have to connect to share data and next, make sure that systems can understand and work with this data when the data is transferred between systems.

In broad terms, we have three different levels of interoperability: the syntax in technology, including the structuring of data, the semantic interoperability, where the data has the same meaning in the different medical protocols, and the pragmatic level of everyday usage of data in practical decision-making.

This is a very simplified explanation of concepts such as **Distributed Data System by Object Management Group (OMG DDS)**. This international standard addresses the real-time publish-subscribe communication for embedded systems by declaring a virtual global data space. In this space, applications can share information through data objects that are defined by an application-defined name called a topic and a key. In other words: DDS allows for real data integration. On top of this global space, DDS supports local object models.

In our case, the DDS domain is the health data space. These data spaces need governance, not only by standards such as OMG DDS but also regulations. One of these regulations is the **European Health Data Space (EHDS)**.

Jeroen Tas, former chief of innovation and strategy at Philips and now a member of the board of directors of European cloud initiative Gaia-X, says about the EHDS: *"We have enormous possibilities with data in the healthcare sector. We can eliminate overdue care, increase capacity, analyze patients, and gain more insight into diseases. But that process is difficult because parties are sometimes sitting on their own data. The market is fragmented. Files, processes, and market parties must be brought together in a secure manner, whereby privacy and identity access are guaranteed."*

Each data space has its regulations defining who is allowed to do what with data. It sounds simple but the legal complexity of it tends to create data silos and not data spaces due to privacy and security concerns. This inhibits innovation.

Each data space or subdomain has its own access rules about which authenticated identities have the authority to do something. The integration happens at the user or user class level. Each person should have a personal environment like they have on their smartphone. Each person has a personal set of apps and devices as systems of engagement. To enable this, we need a clear definition of the API and UI.

For our personal space, we can look at a concept that was put forward by internet pioneer Tim Berners-Lee, called SOLID, which stands for social linked data. In essence, SOLID is a development approach that fits the concept of Web 3.0, where users own and/or direct their personal assets such as data. The promise of SOLID is to decouple applications from the data, and it is built completely according to the microservices principles. With this concept, users have complete freedom in where their data is stored and who is allowed to access that data. It's truly a personal data space.

SOLID makes information accessible through microservices. We can apply these principles for health data, using information standards as in the IHE and CIM, specifically ISO 13972:2022, an international standard meaning there are no restrictions when traveling abroad on the availability of data both in syntax and semantics. For the understanding we seek, it's enough to know that the information in the ICF model can be defined with these standards. Although that's difficult, focus should stay on the value and not the standard itself.

Integration along relations

With the understanding of the entities, we can now address the relations themselves to understand integration. First, we define four relations between the providing entities:

- HeX "provided by" micro-enterprises who treat diseases and/or other interventions to improve the health condition, lifestyle, and ability to participate

- Micro-enterprises "using" workflows consistent with the procedures

- Procedures "requiring" information on the medical condition, circumstances, and care provisioning

- Information that "supports" the HeX with the patient record and overarching care plans

Together, they form the health enterprise. Then, we have four relations between the providing and enabling entities:

- Information is "accessed through" microservices, for instance, the apps

- Procedures "build from" microservices, which form the specifications for the systems of record

- User classes "perform roles" in micro-enterprises, which can be care teams or support teams

- Micro-enterprises "performing in" Point-of-care Environments, either remote or on-site

These four relations are critical as a common understanding is required to lead to the contracts and specifications to develop, build, deliver, and maintain the enabling technology. Within, we have six relationships between entities of the enabling system of systems:

- Point-of-care Environments "provide facilities for" user classes. Think of providing workplaces with a smartphone, tablet, PC, or other devices for professionals and smart clinical beds for patients. These can be Internet of Things devices.

- User classes "that access" microservices via the systems of engagement. We learned that this access plays an important role in securing trust in digital healthcare.

- Microservices "realized with" the operations framework.

- Operations framework "connected to" the Internet of Things.

- Internet of Things "used by" user classes and supported accordingly. This usage normally requires a display and buttons or other I/O devices, the physical part of systems of engagement.

- Internet of Things "placed in" Point-of-care Environments. This includes the logistics to deliver and install these facilities.

The last two are the value relations. Those are the touchpoints on the journeys and OODA loop excursions where the Moments of Truth take place:

- Procedures "resulting in" journeys of episodes of care with touchpoints

- Journeys "executed by" user classes of people and devices with authorization for the specific roles under certain circumstances in the activities in the touchpoints

These two relations of executing itself and the results from execution, bring everything together and form the touchstone of healthcare performance.

This completes all entities and relations in a structure that we will use later on. By following the relation arrows along the entities, for each actual real-life touchpoint, the following questions can be asked: who does what and why? Where and when? What rules should be followed? How can these questions can be explored with all stakeholders? The users can tell their stories along these structured relations and entities. The operators and developers understand these structured stories to plan the initial functionality and subsequent improved iterations based on the new stories from experience.

Now that we have discussed how to tell stories to each other, we should have a closer look at the governance of the community. That's what the next section is about.

Applying SSP, governance, and operations

We have to set up governance, which has to follow the development of networked care from case management to directed care. Here, we will see what has to be set up for each type of networked care:

- Case management starts, for example, with insurance companies having a role in kickstarting virtual or ad hoc networks and making sure communication is clear between the care providers and that coordination for case management is defined. Case management can be enabled to be self-management or management by the next of kin, a case manager from the municipality, or one of the healthcare providers. The governance is embedded in service levels specified in the contract and certifications from an independent body. For IT operations, we refer to the TECOM model for the availability of digital equipment. We can call this Ops "light." The direct per-user cost of the platform is included in the reimbursement tariffs.

- For stepped care, we need a formal collaboration working toward a certain health condition – in our example, to create a seamless journey toward mobility. Stepped care reduces the claims needed. Here, the usability of the platform in the stepped care processes becomes the target. For operations, the comprehensive eTOM, from which TECOM is derived, is suitable to govern the complexity. Maturity assessments and **Total Cost of Ownership** (**TCO**) are the **Key Performance Indicators** (**KPIs**) for the platform.

- Cooperating in integrated care has the benefit of reaching for shared savings on healthcare costs and dividing the savings among the participants. Therefore, eTOM has to be adapted to include specific care, resulting in Ops4Care. The platform must provide a utility with a **Return on Investment** (**ROI**) on the shared savings via a balanced scorecard in the integrated care operations.

- Finally, directed care becomes possible if the whole population can be managed to maximize the economic value with the value board. Health becomes a manageable investment in the population. The entire DevOps4Care process ensures innovation and person-centered delivery. The **Adjusted Clinical Group** (**ACG**©) from John Hopkins or other algorithms are used to predict and anticipate which resources are needed for a healthy population.

Note

For more details on the ACG by John Hopkins, we cordially refer you to `https://www.hopkinsacg.org`.

The following table provides an overview of the governance of the TEC platform:

	Case management	Stepped care	Integrated care	Directed care
Value	Reimbursement	Health	Lifestyle	Participation
Value board	Insurance company / Purchasing department	Collaboration steering group	Cooperation committee	Community representation
Quality management	Service levels and certification, direct cost	Maturity assessment, TCO	BSC, ROI	Population ACG, economics
Financing	Per user	Per use	Shared savings	Population management
Operations	TECOM (availability)	eTOM (usability)	Ops4Care (utility)	DevOps4Care (revenue)

Table 9.5 – Overview TEC platform governance

Governance is about community building and it is here where the panarchy principles apply. The speed of community building will set the order and pace, not the technology. Given the complexity, it will take time to build a common understanding and navigate the panarchy dynamics. It takes time to learn to tell clear stories to each other.

> **Note**
>
> A way to start governance and community building for a platform is using the Contract for the Web from, yet again, Tim Berners-Lee. A good exercise would be to adapt this yourself for healthcare. More information can be found at `https://contractfortheweb.org`.

Summary

In this chapter, we have learned that a common understanding of interoperability and integration can be achieved by using reference models to identify the relations to be used in stories to the operators and developers. We have addressed integration and interoperability as the two critical issues that we must solve in a complex ecosystem. That requires understanding the technology, as well as the interaction of multi-disciplinary teams that work together from a care perspective. It's all part of TiSH and DevOps4Care, as we have shown in this chapter.

We also learned how to unbundle and rebundle organizations in TEC and supporting teams using OODA loops to establish networked care with ever more value, ultimately for the patient but clearly addressing the roles that all stakeholders have in networked and integrated care. We learned how to implement these care models in feasible and defined steps.

Lastly, we demonstrated how to arrange and grow the governance model to ensure operability. We explored several technology domains, such as AI, Internet of Things, and data, and for additional learning on these topics, we kindly refer to the titles in the *Further reading* section. In the next section, we will learn how to perform assessments using TiSH, as a starting point to grow maturity in healthcare transformation.

Further reading

In this chapter, we mentioned a number of frameworks and initiatives. This section gives links to more information:

- Data Distribution Service by the Object Management Group: `https://www.dds-foundation.org`
- Gaia-X: `https://gaia-x.eu/what-is-gaia-x/about-gaia-x/`
- European Health Data Space: `https://health.ec.europa.eu/ehealth-digital-health-and-care/european-health-data-space_en`
- SOLID: `https://solidproject.org/about`
- IHE: `https://www.ihe.net`

Part 3: Applying TiSH – Architecting for Transformation in Sustainable Healthcare

After finishing this part, you will have learned how to apply TiSH, OODA, and DevOps4Care through real-world examples, step by step. In the forthcoming chapters, we will bring it all to life.

The following chapters will be covered under this section:

- *Chapter 10, Assessments with TiSH*
- *Chapter 11, Planning, Designing, and Architecting the Transformation*
- *Chapter 12, Executing the Transformation*

Assessments with TiSH

Our career in transforming healthcare is really taking shape. It's time to tell MoM TiSH how it is going.

We will explore the elements that we need to assess and how to perform assessments, all in good preparation for the transformation. For this, maturity models are introduced with emphasis on the approach of the **Industry 4.0 Maturity Index**. This combines multiple maturities on different themes such as technology, culture, organization, and collaboration to devise a program of activities to allow networked care to grow toward maturity in a balanced way.

We will learn what maturity is, how to get a joint picture of the current maturity, and how to translate that to the next coordinated steps. With this, we can make the transformation into an actionable program of projects and apply it in our daily practice.

In this chapter, we're going to cover the following main topics:

- Understanding and defining maturity assessments with TiSH
- Performing assessments
- Maturity-driven program management

Understanding and defining the assessments with TiSH

Maturity models are one instrument to plan or influence transformation, by determining where we stand today and where we want to go. The most well-known maturity model is the **Capability Maturity Model** (**CMM**), which basically defines at what level organizations have matured in software development. However, CMM is used more widely than just in software development, and frankly, the principles of CMM are quite commonly used in other terrains as well.

As you can see in the following diagram, the TiSH staircase has been inspired by it.

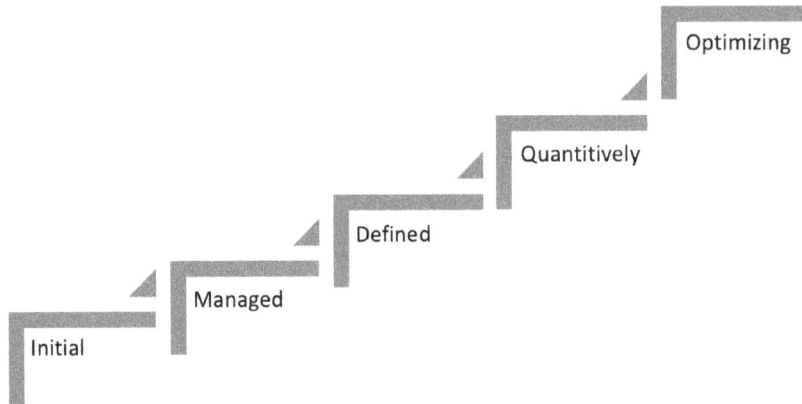

Figure 10.1 – The five levels of the CMM

The basic level of the maturity model is **Initial**. At this level, processes are not well defined. Outcomes are unpredictable since processes are poorly controlled and highly reactive. The next level in CMM is **Managed**. In CMM, it means that processes are defined per project but still very reactive. Even worse, since they are defined per project, organizations constantly need to reinvent the wheel for new projects. Processes are not generic.

The next level is **Defined** where processes are proactive and applicable for organizations and, in our case, collaborations as a whole. The final levels are **Quantitively** managed where processes are controlled, and outcomes are measured and ultimately continuously **Optimizing**. At this highest level, organizations and collaborations can focus on value creation.

In short, organizations start with ad hoc, uncontrolled processes and, via repeatable processes, eventually grow their maturity to proactive, measurable, and foremost predictable outcomes that can be used to continuously improve these outcomes – first within the organization and then adding value in collaboration and cooperation with others.

Maturity models come in all sorts, including models for security and DevOps processes. Systems engineering has also been put into the **Software Engineering Institute Capability Maturity Model Integration** (**SEI CMMI**) framework, which also follows the five levels covering how well the capabilities are developed to engage in the engineering of complex systems.

Many generic models on digital transformation have been developed as well, such as Gartner's Analytics Maturity Model and many more under the collective name of **Digitalization Maturity Model (DMM)**. Specific to healthcare, the **Healthcare Information and Management Systems Society (HIMSS)** developed several models:

- **Adoption Model for Analytics Maturity (AMAM)**

- **Continuity of Care Maturity Model (CCMM)**

- **Supply Chain Model (CISOM)**

- **Digital Imaging Model (DIAM)**

- **Infrastructure Adoption Model (INFRAM)**

- **Outpatient Electronic Medical Record Adoption Model (O-EMRAM)**

- **Electronic Medical Record Adoption Model (EMRAM)**

These models are prescriptive frameworks for healthcare organizations to build their digital health ecosystems. **Healthcare Information Management Systems Society (HIMMS)** uses eight-stage (0–7) maturity models that operate as a development roadmap and offers global benchmarking. TiSH, on the other hand, is a conceptual nonprescriptive frame of mind for building a common understanding between stakeholders of medical and social care, health enterprise, business, and technology.

Tip

For more detailed information on these models, refer to `https://www.himss.org/what-we-do-solutions/digital-health-transformation/maturity-models?gclid=CjwKCAjwh-CVBhB8EiwAjFEPGYWSlAdXR-VgHQqDhZmXCT8fKFPZj738u_pRv3CKNtWRjx9oj_tFeRoCPloQAvD_BwE`.

Another example emphasizing the collaboration of organizations in supply networks is the Industry 4.0 Maturity Index, developed by Acatech and also referenced in Vision35 of INCOSE. Acatech looks at the maturity of several structural areas at the same time on the scale of the collaborating and cooperating supply networks. The addition to HIMMS is their integral view on a set of maturities.

Acatech defines four areas with two principles each, by which the Industry 4.0 maturity is determined:

- **Resources**:

  - Digital capability

  - Structural communication

- **Information systems**:

  - Information processing

  - Integration

- **Organizational structures**:

  - Organic internal organization

  - Dynamic cooperation in the network

- **Culture**:

  - Willingness to change

  - Social collaboration

Based on the current capabilities of these areas, organizations can plan their development path of processes and organizational structure to increase the maturity in Industry 4.0. The index itself has six stages of all maturities combined:

- **Computerization**: In our terms, digitization.

- **Connectivity**: For workflows in processes.

- **Visibility**: What is happening, and seeing or observing others in the network.

- **Transparency**: Why it is happening, and understanding.

- **Predictive capacity**: What will happen, and being prepared.

- **Adaptability**: How can an autonomous response be achieved? Self-optimizing.

In TiSH, we have analog seven treads wherein the first equivalent Acatech stage is covered by two treads. We make a distinction in the resources: digital human skills and technical specifications of devices and the capability to use them in the work within teams. At the organization's tread in the TiSH staircase model, we connect the providing teams to each other and with the enabling teams and their systems. Visibility is how well the care provider organization can communicate with the care network about what is happening. Transparency coincides with the need for coordination in stepped care. Predictive capacity is needed to be prepared and control the individual demand for integrated care. Adaptability allows to autonomously respond with the required measures for a healthy and participating population and the individual people therein.

We use, however, in the stage of reasoning and exploring the models we have put forward in the previous chapters to characterize the maturity of the organization and networked care. This is to facilitate the common understanding in a multidisciplinary setting prior to using the formal models in the qualification and specification, as in CAFCR REQS (Customer, Application, Functional, Conceptual, Realization and Reasoning, Exploring, Qualifying, Specifying). Remember *Figure 5.13* for this. As our main purpose is the health experience, we can translate the Industry 4.0 maturity stages for exploring the development path toward the TiSH staircase of *Chapter 1, Understanding (the Need for) Transformation*. Let's recap what we have learned.

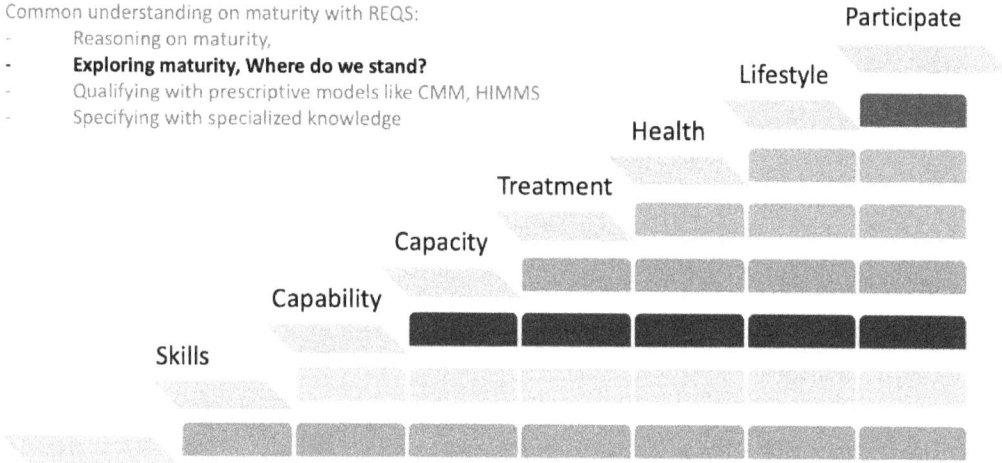

Common understanding on maturity with REQS:
- Reasoning on maturity,
- **Exploring maturity, Where do we stand?**
- Qualifying with prescriptive models like CMM, HIMMS
- Specifying with specialized knowledge

Figure 10.2 – TiSH as the maturity exploration framework

The first tread is about skills and the right devices for one-to-one activities in care delivery. Think of single-task digitization as an eConsult or a medication dispenser. It's about interacting digitally with the Point-of-care.

The second is the teams that learn to work together by informing each other what to do and dividing labor among them based on feedback. Buurtzorg teams are autonomous to divide their labor supported by digital planning and scheduling, or as in real-time *Uber-style* fulfillment without planning, such as the Roamler Care approach.

Thirdly, the organization connects and enables the teams to work on the same Point-of-care together by sharing real-time insights digitally via electronic patient records, or respond to events triggered by social or sensor alarming.

Being on this third tread doesn't mean that there is no **Electronic Patient Record (EPR)** or social alarming in treads one and two. In the first or second tread, the EPR is often used for quality registration purposes to be able to show the quality of care and comply with regulations. The EPR is not much used in the direct interaction with the Point-of-care. In the second tread, it might be used to store the results of questionnaires or retrieve information when preparing for a new interaction, maybe as a result from a social alarm. The difference on thread three is that it's real time.

On the fourth thread, the group of teams acts as single entity, meaning rebundled, to the Point-of-care and digitally visible for the ad hoc care network. They communicate what has happened. The group is part of the case management or performs the role of the case manager itself.

This evolves in the next treads into transparent digital insights in formal Stepped Care collaborations with predictive required capacity, Integrated Care with simulations and algorithms, and Directed Care with adaptable resources autonomously directed from the Point-of-care, all with managed closed loops.

The position on the staircase must be backed by the underlying characteristics, as we have discussed so far in our models. We can group these models into four similar structural areas, each with two principles as two sides of the same medal, recognized in the following:

- **Humans**:

  - Using on one side the health experience stages, from a one-on-one activity to combined distributed care networks, resulting in Directed Care. See *Chapter 3, Unfolding the Complexity of Transformation*.

  - Using on the other side the monetized value staging as given in *Figure 3.4* from individual earnings to outlook on participation. See *Chapter 3, Unfolding the Complexity of Transformation*.

- **Grow**:

  - The size on one side for which the assessment is applicable, including individuals, teams, organizations, collaboration, cooperation, community, and society. See *Chapter 6, Applying the Panarchy Principle*.

  - The planning of growth on the other side as given in *Figure 5.9* from scenarios in campaigns on participation and translation into missions, vision, goals, strategy, tactics, and operations. See *Chapter 5, Leveraging TiSH as Toolkit for Common Understanding*.

- **Digital**:

  - Digitization on one side as put forward in *Table 7.1* and *Table 7.2*, from acting, deciding, orienting, observing, and the loops on observing results, diagnostics, and treatments. See *Chapter 7, Creating New Platforms with OODA*.

  - Complexity on the other side in interoperability and integration from components, subsystems, systems, and engagement systems of systems at tree level, forest level, mission level, and campaign level. Refer to *Chapter 3, Unfolding the Complexity of Transformation* and *Chapter 8, Learning How Interaction Works in Technology-Enabled Care Teams*.

- **Control**:

  - Networking and enabling platforms on one side, from the frontend workplace on the edge, back-office applications, and connectivity to the outside world to communicate, coordinate, control, and command care networks. See *Chapter 9, Working with Complex (System of) Systems*.

  - Governance on the other side, with individuals skilled to work in autonomous TEC teams organized in case management, stepped care, integrated care, and directed care. See *Chapter 9, Working with Complex (System of) Systems*.

These four areas form the sentence *humans grow enabled by digital control* – this sentence is a good reminder of our human measure.

The following table gives an overview of all areas and principles presented in this book. We can identify in each of the seven treads the characteristics of each of these principles.

Each cell of the table can have its own maturity level, but this can very quickly become a meaningless exercise, drowning ourselves in the sheer amount of poorly understood data. We need the overview to gain insight:

Humans							
Health eXperience (HeX)	One-to-one activity	Team with labor division	Teams with support	Visible to a random care network	Transparent to an organized care network	Predictive for an integrated care network	Adaptive to a distributed care network
Value	Earn	Budget	Reimbursement	Reduced claims	Health	Lifestyle	Participate
Grow							
Size	1	10	100	1,000	10,000	100,000	>100,000
Planning	Task	Policy	Strategy	Targets	Vision	Mission	Campaign
Digital							
Digitization	Act	Decide	Orient	Observe	O loop	D loop	T loop
Complexity	Component	System	System of Systems	Tree level	Forest level	Mission level	Campaign level
Control							
Networking	Interact	Process	Connect	Communicate	Coordinate	Control	Command
Governance	Skills	Capability	Capacity	Contract	Collaborate	Cooperate	Community

Legend:

	Deploy		Pilot		Prototype		Idea

Table 10.1 – Maturity board

The maturity has been color-coded with an example of the maturities measured in a qualitative way. Bright green is deployed and blue is piloted, fading via orange for a prototype to light pink in the idea stage. White means that this is currently not a topic. In the next section about performing assessments, we will explain this.

Relating ambition to risk

To establish the position, we can use maturity to set the level of ambition. However, here comes the warning: ambition in achieving maturity can also introduce risks. Stretching to achieve goals set by ambition can lead to frustration in organizations, teams, and individuals, but can also result in failures, impairment, and serious damage where even patients might be severely impacted. For example, you don't want to end up in a situation wherein the security of implants will be compromised. Part of defining the maturity levels is defining the acceptable risk level and introducing proper risk management – proper in this case meaning that human measure and safety are the leading principles.

Proper risk management starts with acknowledging that processes start initially poorly documented, ad hoc, and based on non-integrated policies and systems. The first step to take is to get to repeatable processes that are well defined and can be controlled. As with CMM, the final level in risk management is optimized, where closed-loop processes lead to predictable outcomes and risks can be identified, quantified, and mitigated with strategy and best practices. Only by complying with risk management, organizations, teams, and professionals will we be able to create and work in a coherent digital ecosystem. How do we mitigate this?

We've discussed the content and use of maturity models such as CMM, HIMMS, and Acatech. Again, these models are very formal. For use in a quality system and risk management, this is very useful. For transforming, we need a culture of a more hands-on actionable approach appreciated by people.

Culture is also more expanded in Society 5.0 in Japan: *"A human-centered society that balances economic advancement with the resolution of social problems by a system that highly integrates cyberspace and physical space."* This view is influential on transformation into sustainable healthcare. That's why we utilize maturity in an appreciative cultural approach in reasoning and exploration but still use the valuable insights from Carnegie Mellon, HIMMS, and Acatech.

Our human measure approach uses positive health experience as a merit. For this, the teams who interact with patients or clients and their community must balance the use of technology as an enabler during exploration. How are we going to achieve that balance? That's the topic in the next section.

Performing assessments

Before we dive into the assessments, let's recap some of *Chapter 4, Including the Human Factor in Transformation*, and *Chapter 5, Leveraging TiSH as Toolkit for Common Understanding*. In *Chapter 4, Including the Human Factor in Transformation*, we introduced **Customer Objectives, Application, Functional, Conceptual, Realization (CAFCR)** with the **Requirements (REQS)** layers to turn TiSH into a thinking framework. In *Chapter 5, Leveraging TiSH as Toolkit for Common Understanding*, we introduced the reasoning approach. In fact, the assessments serve a purpose in this reasoning approach. The reasoning gives the assessments meaning in the exploration of specific details.

First, we identify the dominant need or problem as a starting point. The initial need can be to establish what the position is on the TiSH staircase. We look at the CAFCR views on the following:

- Customer objectives, as in individuals digitally interacting with each other using the Activity Triangle to structure stories

- Application requirements on the entities and relationships of the enabling system of systems, using *Figure 9.4* in *Chapter 9, Working with Complex (System of) Systems*

- Functions from actors, sensors, controllers, and use cases creating value through closed OODA-loops with the **Journey Interaction Matrix (JIM)**

- Conceptual decomposition into the entities (refer to *Chapter 9, Working with Complex (System of) Systems*)

- Realization in an enabling system of systems, including an operations framework and defined provisioning entities

The reasoning thread iterations require explorative assessments such as the following three methods, which we will discuss in more detail:

- Qualities checklist to create insights

- Scaling questions to analyze stories and establish facts that deepen insights, next to testing assumptions through simulation in models and measurements of actual use – the evidence backing the stories

- An appreciative inquiry to ask the why, what, how, when, which, where, and other questions to broaden insight

For the integration into the qualities of **Quality Function Deployment (QFD)**, as we defined in *Figure 5.11*, more prescriptive maturity models as sub-methods are needed, such as HIMMS or CMM, to define and extend the reasoning thread. We will not cover that in this book and refer to the sources in the tip given previously and later on in the *Further reading* section.

Qualities checklist for readiness

The next question is how to define the current levels in an organization or determine the readiness for the desired position. A quick scan method for this is by working through a questionnaire. We define five stages in this questionnaire:

- No topic or evidence of it

- Have some ideas (imaginable) worked out in slideware

- Proof of concept in an experimental project (feasible), including a prototype, report, or publication

- Pilot on a small scale (usable, maintainable, and cost structure), subsidized by an organization and/or external funding

- Deployed (applicable, manageable, affordable, and enabling infrastructure in place) with contracted care

The following diagram shows these levels in an innovation chain and associated criteria, which was first introduced by A.W. Mulder, a lecturer at The Hague University of Applied Sciences.

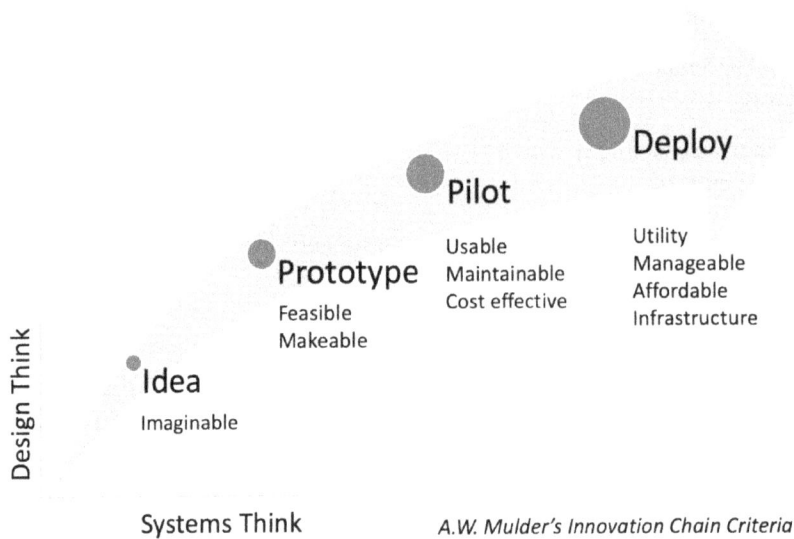

Figure 10.3 – Five stages identified in readiness

For each of the cells, the status can be asked of one or more persons. If they choose a certain level, they must consider how to substantiate this by being able to show evidence of activities. Each cell gets an appropriate color, as shown in *Table 10.1*.

Scaling question assessment

The second method is the use of scaling questions. It's used in therapy and when coaching people and is also suitable to assess the present, past, and future of teams, organizations, and collaborations. It is straightforward by determining the following:

- On which tread, stage, or level do you think the organization stands?
- What has been achieved previously?
- In what situation or circumstance was nothing achieved?
- What was an earlier success?
- What is the next ambition?
- What is ultimately desired?

The following table provides guidance on how to register the preceding questions:

Nothing achieved		Achieved	Current position	Next ambition	Earlier success		Desired
	Foundation of established treads						

Table 10.2 – Scaling question of which TiSH tread an organization is

This scaling question instrument can be used in practice by laying out the eight (0–7) treads on the floor, with each tread about a meter apart, either indoors or outdoors. Now each person can walk the scale and you can observe which position each person in the group takes, indicating where they think the team, organization, or collaboration is at. By exploring together why they have determined the current position, we can establish what has been achieved to date, what earlier success was achieved, and what the next ambition could, should, or must be.

Everyone in the group can ask questions or comment on it. Intervision methods can be useful here. Exploring in a group gives insights into each other's opinions and views. It's a good way to start getting a mutual understanding. The models that we presented earlier are used to project what has been told. This starts the consensus process to reach agreement on the current position and the next step.

This *walking the scale* must be done for all eight characteristics to form the maturity board, as shown in *Table 10.1*, leading to a more comprehensive common understanding and insight.

Appreciative assessments

The third method is the use of appreciative inquiry borrowed from the psychiatric discipline, either in interviews with individuals or groups. It has developed into a powerful transformation tool that can also be applicable outside psychiatry. Here, we apply it to assess the maturities.

It builds on what has already been achieved by individuals, teams, organizations, and collaborations. The scaling questions are good input for the more elaborated appreciative assessments.

The 5Ds of **Define, Discover, Dream, Design, and Deliver** fit nicely into the DevOps4Care process: define the topic or theme, development is the design, ops is delivering, and the dream is the feedback via telling (remember the 4Care steps of experience, value and tell) from the discovery of experience and value in 4Care provisioning. This way, we can make assessments part of DevOps4Care. In fact, the qualities checklist as part of REQs – reasoning, exploring, qualifying and specification – fits in monitor of Ops, and scaling questions are an effective instrument to explore 4Care.

Appreciative assessments go one step further, as they make feedback happen. With feedback, we think again of OODA. And yes, we can express appreciative inquiry in terms of OODA, as shown in the following diagram.

Appreciate the current position and earlier successes, imagine or dream about what could be done, design your future, and create in the ecosystem micro-communities. Combined with self-reflection (Grant), we use OODA to create the loops required for the transformation.

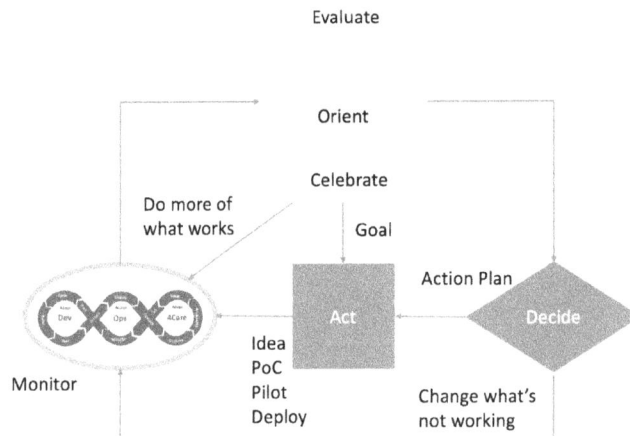

Figure 10.4 – Appreciative assessment and self-reflection

OODA is not only used to model care but also, in Ops, to model the operations, as seen in *Chapter 9, Working with Complex (System of) Systems*, and now the maturity of DevOps4Care itself.

By observing or monitoring the maturity, it is evaluated. Implicit guidance consists of *do more what has worked so far*, changing the goals, or deciding to change *what's not working*. An action plan is made to explore the ideas, build a prototype or conduct a small-scale pilot to test the change before deploying it.

During orientation, every new insight has to be appreciated and celebrated to create a positive attitude to change. This is where the name of the method is derived from: everything that has been done or thought through well is appreciated. The previous methods of scale walking and readiness are the inputs for this method. Again, all eight characteristics must be assessed as different viewpoints on maturity and how it is appreciated.

And of course, we can perform a deep dive with the prescriptive maturity models that we mentioned at the beginning of this chapter. But it's important to maintain a mutual understanding. We can always use TiSH to present the results of these deep dives in a way that resonates with other disciplines and their viewpoints and knowledge.

This brings us to what to do with the results of the reasoning and exploration using assessments. That is the topic of the next section.

We conclude this section with the remark that to establish a common understanding of maturity, a task force should use professionals proficient in using the three assessment methods of a readiness checklist, scaling questions, and appreciative inquiry.

Maturity-driven program management

To engage in transformation, we will use the insights given by the assessment we talked about in the previous section. The question is how to plan the next actionable step from the current position, as concluded in the assessment. We do that by planning the ideation, prototype, pilot, and deployment projects.

We know that development has two sides. It's the maturity and the factors that can inhibit a development path. To stay focused, we have to concentrate on constraining maturity and/or inhibitions. In discussing constraints, we will use Goldratt's **Theory of Constraints** (**TOC**) and keep things actionable.

The takeaway from TOC is to know what bottlenecks are likely to hinder progress. Every system has a limiting factor or constraint. TOC helps with five focusing steps, which, when customized for our transformation, are as follows:

1. Identify the constraining maturity and/or inhibition for the next TiSH tread.
2. Exploit this constraining maturity and/or inhibition.
3. Subordinate everything else to this constraint.
4. Elevate the constraint.
5. Don't stop now and find the next constraint.

We have determined the maturity with the methods introduced in the previous section. What we have not yet done is find the possible inhibitions for the maturity development path.

Let's go back to *Chapter 6, Applying the Panarchy Principle,* where we learned to spot inhibition points in the panarchy. The inhibition points on the ecocycles can be considered bottlenecks. For example, in countries with an aging population, the inhibition point currently is the lack of healthcare personnel. Therefore, we have to make optimum use of the personnel that is available through digitalization. However, the lack of IT personnel creates an inhibition point too in the available technology to enable care.

With this knowledge, we have to make use of what is available in technology and personnel and exploit this as much as possible. We can use the available cloud services and concentrate on using them to eliminate any waste in the care processes and improve the outcomes of their work, maximizing the direct interaction time with patients where the human touch is most needed and automating all other tasks as much as possible.

Transformation of this kind means disruption. Throughout this book, we have advocated unbundling organizations into micro-enterprises and re-bundling them into ecosystem micro-communities. We advise having a look at Geoffrey A. Moore's book *Zone to Win.* Moore defines four zones to create – or facilitate – disruption and to get organizations to start investing and exploring new ways of working. The four zones are shown in the following ecocycle diagram:

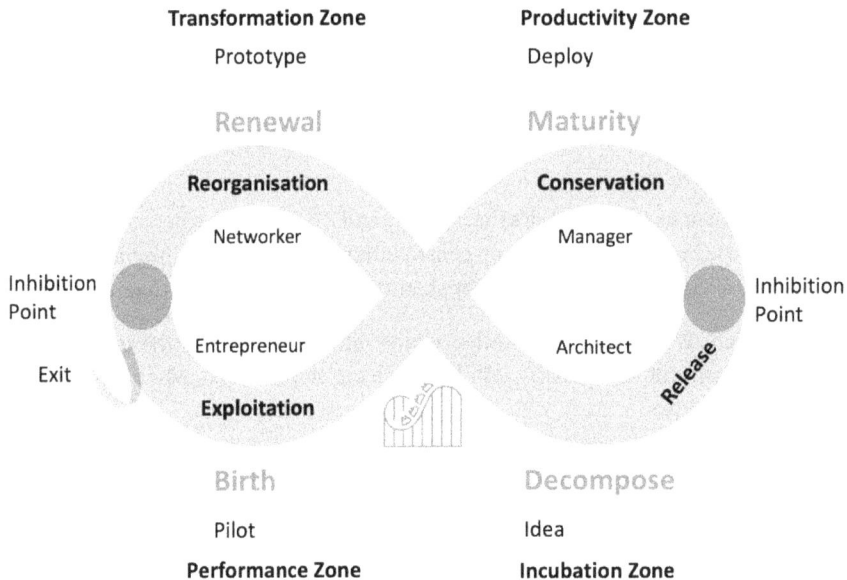

Figure 10.5 – Moore's zones and readiness in the planning ecocycle

The first two zones are the performance and the production zones. These zones aim for sustainment; they basically keep everything the way it is and do not disrupt but change gradually. The big risk here – remember the section where we talked about risk management – is that organizations in these zones will be disrupted from the outside. Other new organizations will invest in new products and services, addressing the changing needs of people's health.

Organizations must get to the disruptive zones, starting with the incubation zone, where these changing needs of patients are explored and new propositions are created. In this incubation zone, the organization purely invests. It's in the transformation zone where these new propositions and forthcoming solutions are prototyped, gaining more traction in the healthcare ecosystem and reaching more patients for feedback.

However, from the transformation zone, organizations will enter the performance zone again at a certain point. In other words, organizations will constantly have to *re-invent* themselves to keep up with changing and ever-increasing demands. This is extremely hard for big organizations with a monolithic architecture. Hence, we must unbundle and re-bundle into agile operating micro-enterprises, supported by a microservices architecture.

The four zones have their own leadership style. If these leadership styles are not addressed and all zones are not executed in parallel by different types of people, the inhibition points will manifest. Planning the ideation, prototypes, pilots, and deployment must be allocated along the teams in the different zones. As incubating, transforming, and (learning to) perform are costly, cooperation with other care providers can start the next step in networked care.

Of course, here we can find a constraint where some organizations are *not letting go* or *not investing* in overcoming inhibition points. Differences in maturity can be the reason for this.

On the collaboration scale, one organization can become a bottleneck. Again, the focus is on utilizing this organization and elevating this constraint by either a different division of labor and/or one organization learning about the other organization.

To recap: program management enables projects in the four different zones to address the identified lowest maturity and inhibition points, all with the purpose of building the two sides of the following:

- The health experience **Ecosystem Micro-Community** (EMC) around every individual – the HeX at the points of care along the touchpoints of the journey

- The solution ecosystem micro-community to deliver medical and social care in some form of networked care

The terms experience and solution ecosystem micro-communities are used in the Rendanheyi-model to distinguish between the care-facing micro-enterprises and the enabling micro-enterprises. In the next chapter, we will elaborate on this.

In an organization, there are always one or more teams who are motivated to try something else. Take one of these teams to incubate new ideas and give them room to transform themselves on a small scale. Their example can be used to pilot a new approach with other teams, and after performance is proven, the rest of the organization or collaboration can follow. With this, the variation in maturity across teams can be put to good use. However, they have to take into consideration what the transformation of all teams will cost in time and resources.

Start small and learn to grow the maturity of the rest of the organization. This is true for building health experience ecosystem micro-communities and for enabling ecosystem micro-communities. To avoid that for every single health experience different enabling systems are developed, which is unsustainable, it has to build on the foundation of the cloud with its generic services.

We mentioned the constraint of the lack of enough IT workers. Cooperation on this with other care providers in the community is a way to start working on the shared services platform and avoid reinventing the wheel in each organization and every health experience. Here, we embrace the cloud strategy. Let's explore this cloud foundation.

Data and applications will have to be hosted somewhere and the way to go is in cloud environments. Organizations might host their own apps and data or use data coming from various sources. Organizations will also use **Software as a Service** (**SaaS**) applications that are hosted in various environments. This landscape is what we call multi-cloud. Make no mistake: almost every organization is already multi-cloud-oriented. They might use Microsoft Office 365, Salesforce, or other **Enterprise Resource Planning** (**ERP**) applications, and data connected to diagnostic equipment, or even **Electronic Patient Data** (**EPD**) that is hosted in cloud environments.

All of this must be operated and managed. It becomes even more complex when organizations develop their own applications using DevOps methodologies, including **Continuous Integration and Continuous Deployment** (**CI/CD**) software pipelines. Organizations must *grow* their maturity in operating these complex environments in order to enable professionals and patients to work with the systems.

In maturity models for multi-cloud governance, we focus on pillars or scaffolds, following the best practices of cloud adoption frameworks that are issued and maintained by major public cloud providers such as Microsoft Azure, AWS, and **Google Cloud Platform** (**GCP**). These pillars contain the following:

- Cost optimization
- Security and compliancy
- Utilization and scaling of resources
- Automation

These frameworks are guidance in moving systems to the cloud and transforming applications and data in the cloud in a way that allows cloud resources to be optimized. **Cloud adoption frameworks (CAFs)** typically start by defining a strategy, then planning for transition and transformation, and finally governing and managing resources – literally taking an organization by the hand in transition and transformation. The strength lies in connecting processes, services, products, and organizations with supporting (cloud) technology, resulting in increased operational efficiency.

> Tip
> The CAFs of Azure and AWS can respectively be found on `https://azure.microsoft.com/en-us/overview/cloud-enablement/cloud-adoption-framework/` and `https://aws.amazon.com/professional-services/CAF/`.

As every organization has to do this, it's a great opportunity to start collaborating and cooperating on the solution enabling side. This brings focus to the operational healthcare activities of the **Technology-Enabled Care (TEC)** teams.

Let's use an example to illustrate this.

We will use *Table 10.1* and now explain the colors of the cells. This care provider has made an assessment with the scaling questions and has concluded that the lowest maturity is the digital area, in digitization and complexity, digitization scores orient level in regards to complexity, where only a prototype has been made to observe the real-time circumstances of the patient. A pilot is underway to have a better overview of the whole complex application landscape to turn it into a consistent system of systems.

The next step is to go for remote monitoring of patients at home. Some experience has been gained in a pilot conducted on integrated care in a consortium. This was a subsidized project that ended last year. Activity trackers and vital sign measurements were part of the project. However, another organization of the consortium provided these.

The insurance company did a pilot on lowering costs in this project. An experiment was conducted to build a prototype to receive the monitoring data directly in the EPR. This experiment failed, but the project was considered a success, as it increased knowledge and common understanding.

The conclusion was that more investments are needed in digitization to be able to observe patients in real time. The bottleneck is that although IT operations are sufficient, they lack the development capacity.

The organization is now discussing whether to invest in development. The inhibition is that it is unclear what the consequences are in terms of value. Reduced claims read as less income for the organization.

It is decided to do a more comprehensive appreciative assessment and make a plan for the mid to long term for the transformation, in not only being able to do remote monitoring but also to investigate collaboration with other care providers and the local government responsible for social care.

In the next chapter, we will explore this further and apply all that we have learned so far.

Summary

In this chapter, we learned what maturity models are and how we can use them to define the maturity level of organizations and teams, and also how to set an ambition to reach the next level. In order to define maturity, we must do assessments. Basically, we should know where we're coming from if we want to determine where we are going – the very essence of any transformation. We learned to use the models in assessments from a checklist, scaling questions, appreciative assessments, and how to plot results on prescriptive maturity models such as CMM and HIMMS.

We learned how to look at maturities of different aspects and sizes to plan for a program of transformation projects. We can define actions to identify the inhibition points and utilize them as much as possible. As a result, we can make a balanced program of ideation, prototypes, pilots, and large-scale deployment projects.

In the final section, we introduced the ecosystem micro-communities and learned how to motivate these to move through various performance zones, continuously improving services and eventually providing better, sustainable healthcare by making use of shared services and resources, such as cloud technology. In the next chapter, we will further discuss these micro-communities.

Further reading

- *CMMI*: https://www.cmmiinstitute.com/

- *Zone to Win: Organizing to Compete in an Age of Disruption* by Geoffrey A Moore

- *Appreciative Inquiry*: https://positivepsychology.com/appreciative-inquiry-process/

- *Theory of Constraints Institute* by E. Goldratt: https://www.theoryofconstraints.org

- *Industrie 4.0 Maturity Index. Managing the Digital Transformation of Companies – UPDATE 2020*: https://en.acatech.de/publication/industrie-4-0-maturityindex-update-2020/download-pdf?lang=en

Planning, Designing, and Architecting the Transformation

Achievements are building. Results are beyond what MoM TiSH has taught us. Time to start your independent path.

We know where we're coming from, and we know where we're going. But how do we get there? We have learned how to do assessments, and we have defined our goal: sustainable healthcare. Based on these assessments, we have learned how to set up a balanced program with projects on ideation, prototypes, pilots, and deployment with different teams. Now, it's time to start planning the transformation itself.

We will learn how to conceptualize the plans, how to form the teams to execute these plans, and what actions are part of it. Now, how do we empower these teams to execute the transformation?

In this chapter, we're going to cover the following main topics:

- Defining the transformation plan
- Designing with **Technology Enabled Care** (TEC) teams
- Empowering transformation teams

Defining the transformation plan

We ended the previous chapter with an example: a care provider deciding to set up a transformation plan. Simply launching another project does not solve the problems experienced. The urgency calls for a transformation.

The dilemmas they encountered are twofold: the contradiction of collaborating with other care providers, resulting in less revenue, and creating the collaboration in the first place while not having enough development resources to create the digital outreach process for patients in their community. Still, the bottom line is that fulfilling the health needs of the population will be valued. The question is how does this translate into real revenue for the organization? And how does digitalization fit into this equation?

To set up the transformation plan, we can use the transposed maturity board of *Table 10.1*, resulting in the following table, which gives a constructive foundation to measure progress:

Aspect / Tread	HeX	Value	Size	Planning	Digitization	Complexity	Networking	Governance
	Adaptive distributed network	Participate	>100,000	Campaign	T-loop	Campaign level	Command	Community
	Predictive integrated network	Lifestyle	100,000	Mission	D-loop	Mission level	Control	Cooperate
	Transparent organized network	Health	10,000	Vision	O-loop	Forest level	Coordinate	Collaborate
	Visible care network	Reduced Claims	1,000	Targets	Observe	Tree level	Communicate	Contract
	Teams with support	Reimbursement	100	Strategy	Orient	SoS	Connect	Capacity
	Team with labor division	Budget	10	Policy	Decide	System	Process	Capability
	One-to-one activity	Earn	1	Task	Act	Comp.	Interact	Skills

Table 11.1 – The program progress board

We use the four types of projects, ideation, prototyping, piloting, and deployment, to fill any gaps. Each cell can be divided into the different types of care provided if needed to address the different maturities. For the most part, an organization is not equally mature in all departments. For our example care provider, we assume it is.

They use their experience to realize the technical solution for the real-time monitoring of outpatients. The pilot for the coherent application landscape managed as a **System of Systems (SoS)** gave valuable insights into the increased complexity, and the care teams gained experience in the experiment where the inhibition points included frustrating technology and anxiety on how remote monitoring worked – remember the work of Knoster that we discussed earlier in this book.

Talks with the insurance company have made it clear that, in 2 years, the use of remote monitoring will become mandatory. In this case, the program would be as follows:

1. **Project A**: Deployment of a cloud strategy on the application landscape to build the SoS and free up IT personnel

2. **Project B**: Pilot the setting up of the remote monitoring service with the freed-up IT personnel and enable the care personnel to observe patients at home

3. **Project C**: Contracting remote monitoring and deploying remote monitoring

4. **Project D**: Ideation project on the next tread of stepped care

Project A has to be finished before project B can start as the IT personnel has to be freed up first. Both have to be finished in 2 years to be on time for the new contracting of health insurance.

In parallel, the ideation for stepped care can be set up together with other care providers and probably followed by an experimental prototype. That is, provided it does not put a strain on the resources for projects A, B, and C.

By using the maturity models, we have a stronger foundation and better control of the risks. Therefore, we will have more successful projects. So, what should the approach to these projects be? We'll discuss this in the next section.

Micro-communities in the health experience ecosystem

In fact, we start at the bottom and build from there. We start with one or a few patient(s) and improve on one or a few simple tasks and learn from there. Although the program is set up top-down from the campaign for a healthy participating population and the derived mission, vision, targets, and strategy, the realization is the other way around. To avoid the pitfall of internalizing the transformation, we have to look to externalize it from the beginning. As a starting point, we need something to address the changing needs of individual people's health. This approach means that a project can never be started without involving the patient or client and their community.

For that we can find further inspiration in the Rendanheyi concept of **Ecosystem Micro-Communities (EMCs)**, as shown in the following diagram:

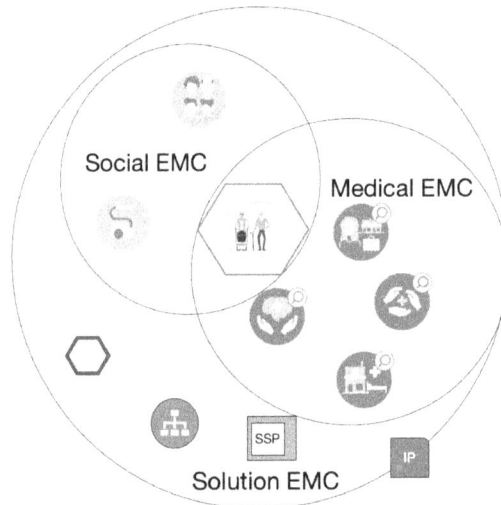

Figure 11.1 – EMCs for organizing health

In the first chapter, we introduced the HeX to incorporate all types of caregivers in the care ecosystem of a person. It's an EMC to create individual health experiences provided by the TEC teams, as discussed in *Chapter 8, Learning How Interaction Works in Technology-Enabled Care Teams*.

At the center, we have the individual or family with their own personal micro-enterprise to arrange their health experience, the HeXagon. In this personal micro-enterprise, we find the next of kin and friends. It's the inner yellow hexagon. This micro-enterprise is supplied by other micro-enterprises for social and medical care. A micro-enterprise equals our TEC teams. Together, they form the Social and Medical EMCs.

The enablers are in the Solution EMC to provide solutions for the care EMC. These are mostly the services from IT, **Human Resources (HR)**, and finance organized in shared services for the EMCs. They are, at the very least, a learning community, and TEC platform (SSP) community, which are governed by the IP Value Board.

This looks like a traditional supply chain, but Rendanheyi is about each employee directly facing the people they attend to, contributing to their health experience, and realizing their own value, too. It's a win-win. Employees are focused on the health experience, using guidelines and guardrails to stay on track to the destination. It's not the other way around, following rigid guidelines and guardrails on fixed journeys.

The way this works is that the patient forms the demand side, which must be understood with a very short *supply* line. The Solution EMC is in direct contact with the care and patients. Translated to DevOps4Care, Ops supports the users of the technology directly.

The challenge is to facilitate the value stages for all involved while creating the health experience. In our example, this is the care provider who wants to solve the dilemma of less revenue in the collaboration and still have the budget for funding technology for the teams and paying salaries. Additionally, the EMC concept is used to remove barriers between micro-enterprises by focusing on the end users of all the combined services.

Because the (potential) patient is the owner of its HeX micro-enterprise, the TEC team of the Social and Medical EMCs is focused on improving health, supported by the enabling teams in the Solution EMC. This evolves along the structures of the micro-enterprises described in *Chapter 9, Working with Complex (System of) Systems*, introducing even more integration into networked care:

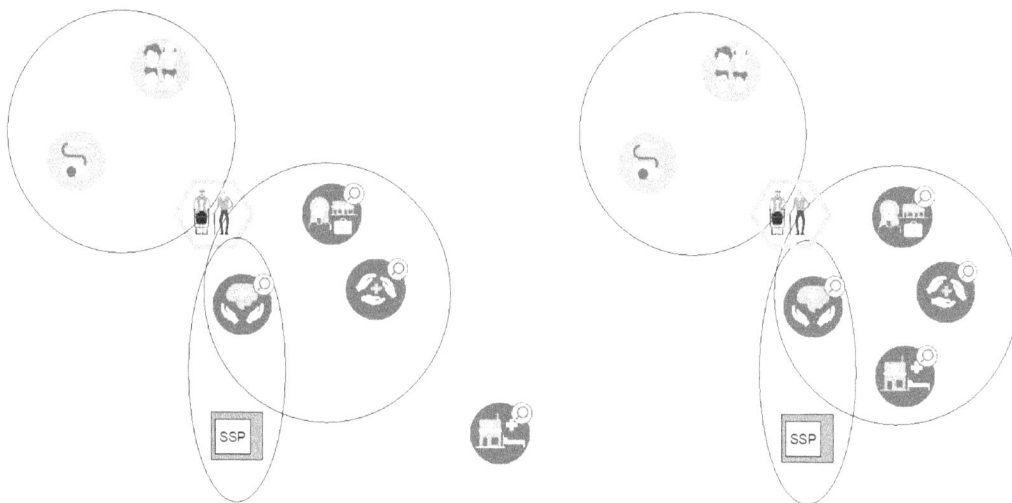

Figure 11.2 – Starting the evolution of networked care from the initial to the first stage

In the preceding figure, our example care provider is still outside the care EMC during the initial stage. The question is how to fit it into the EMC in the first stage.

The governance mentioned in *Table 9.1* guides the access to the EMCs to serve the individual HeX micro-enterprises via the Value Board. Any organization can offer an evidence-based proposition to the Value Board and show how they can contribute to the health experience. Depending on the networked care tread of case management, stepped care, integrated care, or directed care, this is the insurance company, collaboration steering group, cooperation committee, or community representation:

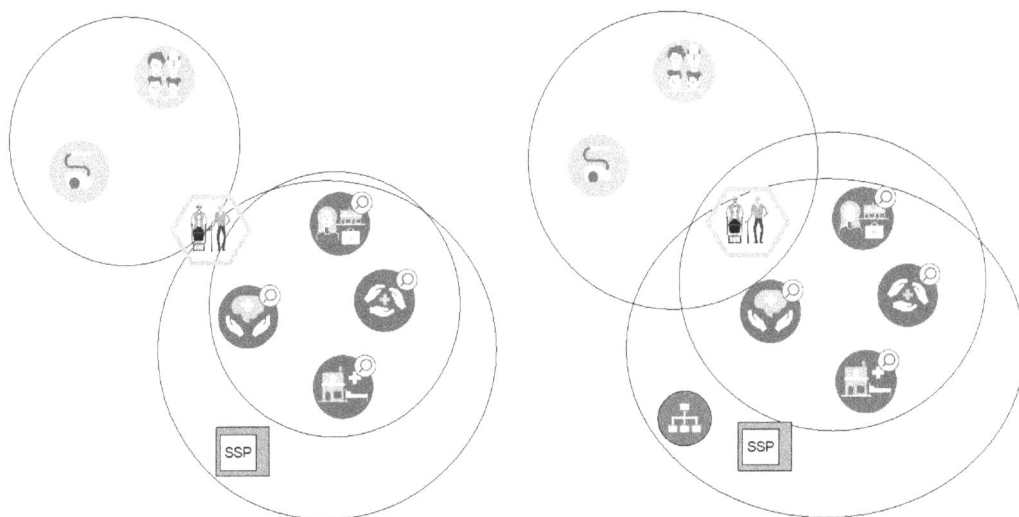

Figure 11.3 – The evolution of networked care in the second and third stages

Once in the EMC, our care provider joins, in the second stage, forces with other care providers making use of the Solution EMC's enabling of cloud services and remote monitoring. Projects A and B are now executed much quicker, and the care provider can focus on the health experience itself. This increases the chance of the successful execution of project C.

The third stage is to align with the social caregivers. This stage is investigated in project D.

The emergence of health experience EMCs from a patient's view

A person starts their personal HeX micro-enterprise by building it from daily life. Sports or other physical activities might be used for prevention but also friends and family who can help when assistance is required. This is informal. Usually, a GP, dentist, physiotherapist, and pharmacist will join the care EMC. Alongside this setup, supporting technology is used: email, chat, social media, and portals for making appointments or ordering repeat prescriptions and looking up medical history with the convenience of smartphones or tablets. The use of an activity tracker or smartwatch is becoming more common. Gadgets such as Wi-Fi-connected toothbrushes and a plethora of health apps are also available.

The personal HeX grows into an ad hoc care EMC, but at a certain point, this develops into networked care starting with case management. Any care provider's question should be how to connect to the care EMC and become part of it.

So, for our example care provider in project B, it's clear that its remote monitoring service has to fit into the health experience, and this orchestration needs to fit into some collaborative TEC platform with other care providers. This seems to be a daunting task. Complexity is not on the list of invitees, but it's there. Here, the **Minimum Viable (or Valuable) Product (MVP)** approach comes to the rescue. Challenge a team to find the lead users from the community, understand their needs, and start improving by defining a first MVP.

> Tip
>
> For an extensive example of how to build a community in general, we recommend the resources on the Community Canvas website at `https://community-canvas.org/#get-started`.

Leveraging the power of small

The goal of this example is to monitor the patient remotely. Based on what has been observed with remote monitoring, a decision is made on how to act. This departs from a scheduled check-up in the clinic and can directly lead to a referral to a mobile nurse or physiotherapist outside the organization, but within the care EMC, for a follow-up. It is expected this will increase the health experience at a lower cost.

The wrong way is to select a product, implement it, and start working with it. This will take the better part of a year, and when deploying many things, it easily gets out of hand, inevitably leading to a bad reputation for the transformation as a whole.

Another way is to select a patient who might already have some ideas about why the remote monitoring could be beneficial: the lead users. With these lead users, experience is built. First, do a paper check of the idea with a few patients, then a prototype with some more, then a pilot, and finally the deployment. The first two steps of ideation and prototype can be done without the strong involvement of IT who will be busy with project A. Only the existing systems are used.

In the ideation step, the check-up is scheduled as normal, but now a nurse will visit the patient at home just before the appointment and check on the condition using portable equipment and decide, together with the patient, whether to go to the scheduled appointment or to shift it to another time. The equipment can be for vital signs, wound checking, or a questionnaire – things that are normally executed at the clinic. The benefit for the patient's health experience is not having to go to the clinic if not needed. Of course, this isn't cost-effective for the care provider yet. This is ideation in the incubation zone.

The second step is ensuring the patient gets the equipment to use at home, either delivered by package delivery or taken when visiting the clinic to get final instructions. This time, the nurse is calling just prior to the scheduled check-up to see what the measurements are and a decision is made on whether to come to the clinic or to refer the patient to another care provider in the EMC. This is the prototype or transformation zone in which the new procedure is tested.

The third step is to let the patient send the measurements to the nurse via secure email. This avoids having to integrate the measuring device into the EPR. The patient does not have to wait for a call from the nurse. Only when the measurements are not satisfactory will the nurse send a message via email with the next step, either an appointment or a referral. This will include a notification to the preferred referral party of the care EMC. The process is adapted in the EPR to have conditional appointments, but no systems integration takes place. This is the pilot in the performance zone.

The final step is to check all the characteristics to see whether all is clear in terms of the requirements for the development of the systems integration and deployment. In the meantime, the application landscape is transferred to the cloud in project A with not only the benefit of freeing up the IT personnel but also the extra security and possibility to make use of the standard IoT and analytics functionality of the cloud.

Now, a selection can be made for a remote monitoring solution with the experience gained in the first three zones. The solution is to use the knowledge of another care provider in the EMC. A collaboration is set up to have a joint platform to facilitate cross-organization processes. This solves the constraint in development capacity in another way.

Connecting the remote monitoring equipment to the EPR is made very easy. The organization is ready for contracts with health insurance reimbursement in the productivity zone, project C.

In discussion with the other care providers regarding the need for coordination around the same person, omniversal care is noticeable. A joint vision that the patients get a seamless service from all care providers emerges. Project D is born to investigate a joint program. The whole program uses a similar approach to the following diagram:

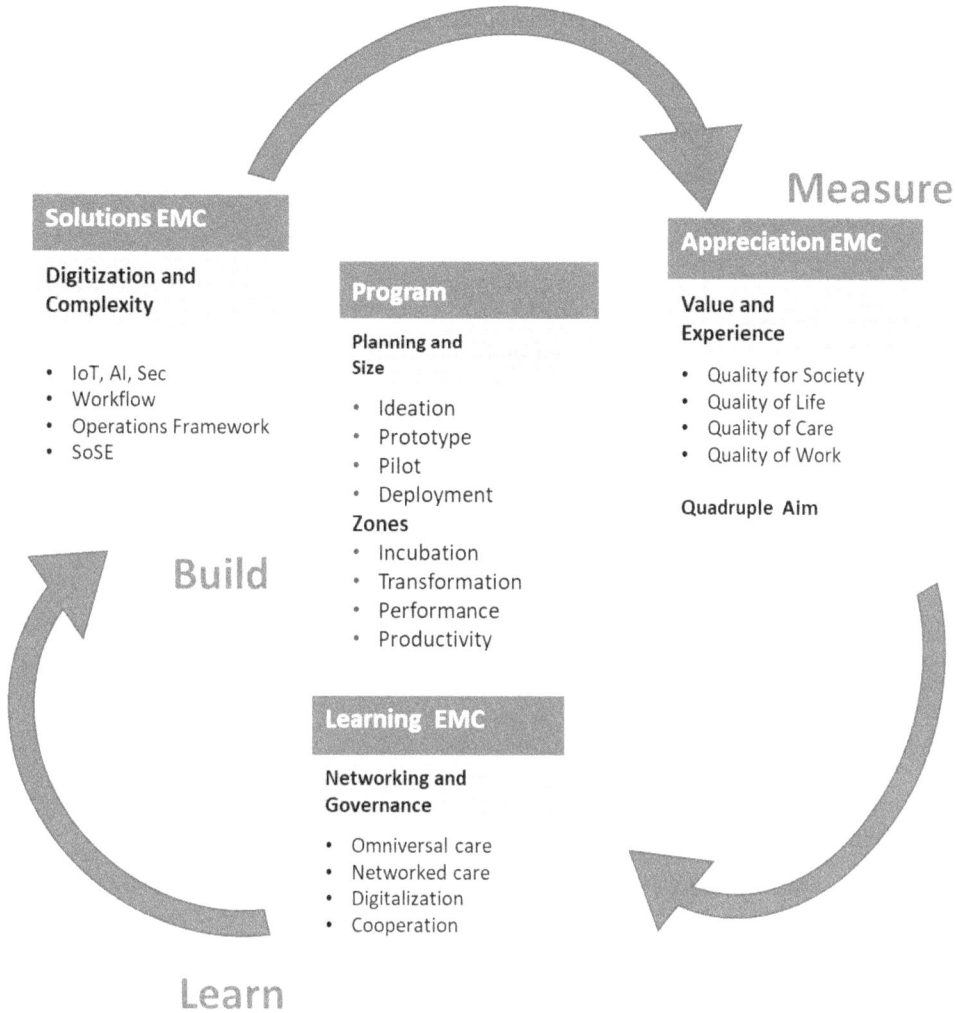

Solutions EMC

Digitization and Complexity

- IoT, AI, Sec
- Workflow
- Operations Framework
- SoSE

Program

Planning and Size

- Ideation
- Prototype
- Pilot
- Deployment

Zones

- Incubation
- Transformation
- Performance
- Productivity

Appreciation EMC

Value and Experience

- Quality for Society
- Quality of Life
- Quality of Care
- Quality of Work

Quadruple Aim

Measure

Build

Learning EMC

Networking and Governance

- Omniversal care
- Networked care
- Digitalization
- Cooperation

Learn

Figure 11.4 – Setting up a program with the Learn, Build, and Measure cycle

In general, we recommend setting up a program with the learn, build, and measure cycle as used for MVPs. The preceding figure shows this MVP cycle including the transformation aspects and main topics within it. To make it actionable, communities for learning, building, and measuring are set up, feeding each other and other care and solution EMCs in the project activities of the program.

Another way to use zoning and project types in maturity-driven program management is to look up the stairs from the current position on the TiSH staircase and plan a deployment for the next tread, a pilot on the tread after that, a prototype on the third tread, and ideation for the fourth.

In our example, this translates into a possible joint program resulting from project D:

- Deployment of case management; one short term
- Pilot on stepped care; short- to mid-term
- Prototype on integrated care; mid-term
- Ideation of directed care; long-term

This will give you time to build the maturities required when needed and build a common understanding with the communities. As with normal education, it takes years to learn. Refer to *Chapter 5, Leveraging TiSH as Toolkit for Common Understanding*, for more information on how to build up the models.

The learn, build, and measure cycle shows the progress in the maturity of all teams and organizations in the communities; therefore, it offers a balanced way to grow together toward sustainability.

Let's take a look at how to apply this to the transformation.

Designing with TEC teams

The transformation itself is led by the members of the TEC teams working as micro-enterprises. These teams will cycle through the learn, build, and measure cycle to drive the design process for the enabling technology. So, looking at *Figure 11.4*, what are important topics to learn, build, and measure?

The main learning topics are listed as follows:

- Omniversal care, including a common understanding between social and medical care and the possibilities of technology, is one of the challenges ahead
- The different forms of networked care; case management, stepped care, integrated care, and directed care
- Digitalization from the act to the treatment loop, including the use of AI algorithms
- Cooperation with other teams in teams of teams to enable systems innovation into sustainable healthcare

The main design topics are listed as follows:

- Systems including IoT, AI, and security realized in **Identity and Access Management** (**IAM**)
- Workflows not only within the organization but also across the EMC and for the operations framework for securing the availability of enabling solutions
- The TEC platform for the shared services built with the **System of Systems Engineering** (**SoSE**)discipline

For the main measuring topics, we have coined the term "quadruple aim" to which the value stages are related. They consist of the following:

- Level of quality for society in terms of participation, cost of care, and sustainability

- Quality of life in terms of health and lifestyle

- Quality of care provided in treatment and other interventions

- Quality of work for anyone involved, including job satisfaction and the appreciation of volunteers

Every cycle in every zone or project type will address these topics in some form. By continuously doing so, the common understanding will grow and, alongside that, so will the success of the transformation. Common understanding is a success factor for the transformation.

Now we will discuss three concepts, addressing each topic to be considered in real-world projects in terms of what to concentrate on in learning, designing what to build, and appreciating what is or has to be measured:

- Cooperation in digital omniversal networked care

- The TEC platform for integration in the community

- The quadruple aim for sustainable healthcare

Cooperation in digital omniversal networked care

One principle in omniversal care is the combination of medical and social care. Learning to understand the power of this combination is an important step toward sustainable healthcare.

First, we will talk about the differences in approaches that are commonly taken, followed by why that combination can benefit the health experience. The first approach is problem-oriented medical care. Indeed, this is about curing or recovering from a disease, the problem. The other approach is solution-oriented social care, which is about the solution to implement given a health or lifestyle problem. In real life, it is not that exclusive, but it serves the purpose of our understanding.

We will briefly discuss the two representative models for each approach, the **Clinical Reasoning Cycle** (**CRC**) for the medical problem approach and **Solution-Focused Therapy** (**SFT**) for the social solution approach.

In the following diagram, we show both models mapped on OODA to make the translation for the digitization steps easier:

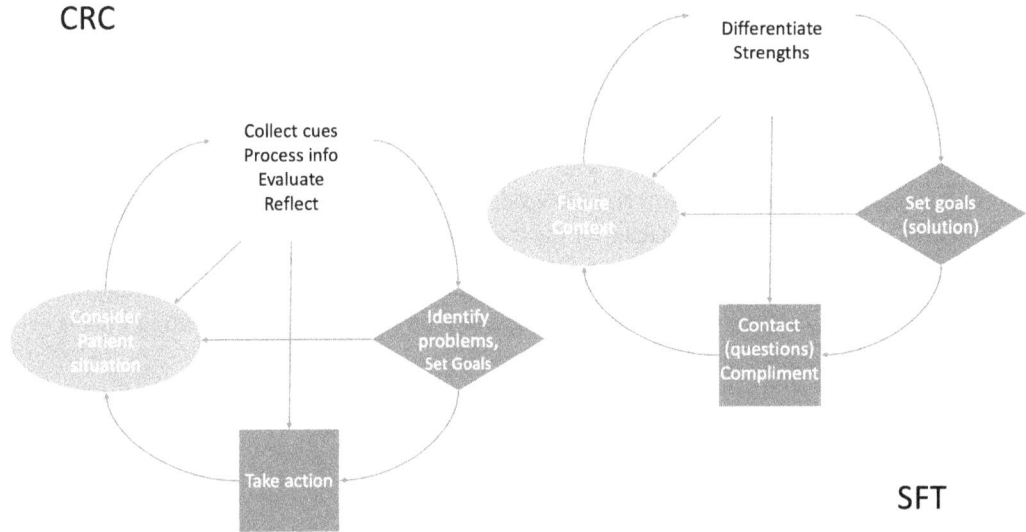

Figure 11.5 – CRC and SFT mapped onto OODA

The CRC has eight phases, consisting of the following:

- Consideration of the patient's situation requiring observation
- Collecting cues from the gathered information
- Processing information and analyzing this with past experiences to predict an outcome
- Identifying problems/issues by synthesizing facts and deciding on the problems
- Establishing goals on the desired outcome for the treatment
- Taking action by choosing the steps needed to meet the patient's treatment goals
- Evaluating the outcomes
- Reflecting and learning to achieve a better outcome, and understanding what should be avoided in similar occurrences in the future

This CRC will facilitate problem-solving and decision-making to provide the best care. Knowing about past health episodes and understanding the problem are key.

SFT was developed by Steve de Shazer and Insoo Kim Berg and is all about finding solutions rather than identifying and eliminating the problem, focusing on addressing what clients want to achieve. By using short interactive interventions including miracle questions, exception questions, coping questions, and scaling questions, they achieved remarkable results. See the following tip for further reading. This approach is very similar to OODA.

Mapped on the OODA steps, this gives the following:

- Make contact so that the observation can commence

- Current context and future wishes are observed

- Orientation on strengths and differentiation on possible solutions

- Set goals for the future

- Above all, act by asking the miracle, exception, coping, and scaling questions

- Make compliments while acting

> **Tip**
>
> More detailed information on CRC can be found in this publication: Levett-Jones, T., Hoffman, K., Dempsey, Y., Jeong, S., Noble, D., Norton, C., et al. (2010). *The 'five rights' of clinical reasoning and educational model to enhance nursing students' ability to identify and manage clinically 'at risk' patients*. Nurse Education Today, 30(6), 515-520.
>
> For an actionable introduction to SFT, we recommend Cauffman, LL. and Dierhof, K., *Solution-focused coaching - seven simple steps to solutions in coaching*, Brave New Books, ISBN:9789402134971

Bringing social and medical care together in the past, present, and future is done by relating it to the ICF model. This will help us to reason and explore how these two interact. In the following diagram, the approaches are linked:

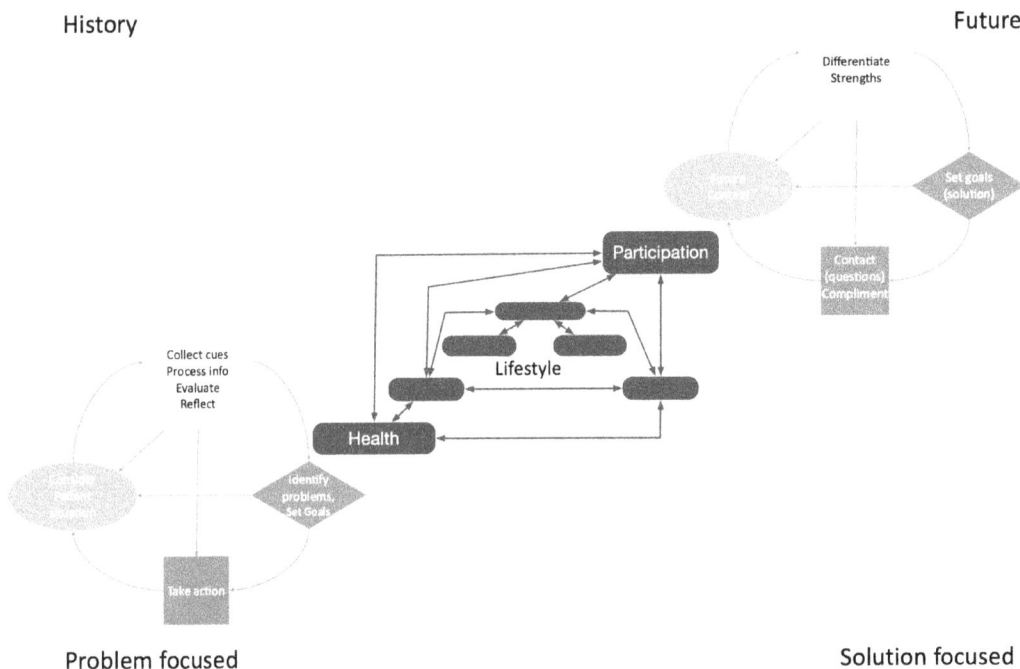

Figure 11.6 – Two complementary approaches to the health experience

CRC is approaching it from the health problem side and SFT from the participation side. Both have in common the circumstances in the environment including lifestyle.

The analyses using AI algorithms consider all factors to find the optimum balance in activities in terms of the health and participation goals. This is also the basis of the INCA model that we discussed in *Chapter 1, Understanding (the Need for) Transformation*.

Indeed, the coordination between the two approaches becomes more important in the highest treads of TiSH. Semantic interoperability and integration are human things; however, the platform has to facilitate all of these different actors to be able to cooperate. The ICF model can help with this by addressing which perspective is being communicated regarding the patient. The systems of intelligence have to be able to process both types of approaches and data.

The TEC platform for integration in the community

Mentioning systems of intelligence involves talking about the TEC platform itself, the second concept to connect the different organizations involved in the community. For each type of networked care, more functionality will be productive. Next to the systems of intelligence, the systems of engagement and systems of record are also impacted. The complexity will increase from the tree level, forest level, and mission level to, eventually, the campaign level.

One way to build a TEC platform is to set up a micro-enterprise for each community consisting of a complement of other micro-enterprises for a full service of the roles and processes defined in the engagement entities, as explained in *Chapter 9, Working with Complex (System of) Systems*. This complement is facing the care EMC and is responsible for delivering the agreed shared services for the micro-community. Operational interoperability and integration are the main tasks to facilitate healthcare provisioning as a starting point and to enable the EMC to continuously improve on their tasks.

The TEC platform adds to the functionality provided by the usually siloed systems of the different organizations. It augments the communication between the care providers and the patients. Therefore, the IT departments of healthcare organizations can become a part of the complement and start the rebundling process.

Now, we will discuss the main functions of each type of networked care.

For case management, it is important that the community knows who is doing which action. Simple messaging and access to applications via a common IAM will enable the necessary communication.

An ecogram is useful here to define the micro-community. For every patient, an ecogram enables you to know who is involved in the patient's micro-community and in which capacity, that is, informal care, social care, and medical care. With this ecogram, every actor in the network knows who else is involved and how to contact them.

Another functionality that is useful at this stage is an agenda where all the planned contact moments from all caregivers can be seen. The benefit to the patient is that joint planning can make it easier to avoid any *traffic jams* of caregivers at the front door. Speaking of front doors, controlling physical access via a smart lock controlled by the IAM function can improve the safety of the patient at home.

For stepped care, decisions have to be coordinated as to who has to execute the next action. Here, cross-organizational workflows will have to be enabled by the TEC platform connecting the systems of engagement of the care providers. Here, solutions such as Microsoft Power BI Report Builder, ServiceNow, Zapier, SAP, Oracle, or other integration and workflow platforms can be useful for creating a better health experience so that the patient is attended to at the right place by the right provider in a seamless experience.

A lot of the communication that is needed in case management must be replaced by workflow rules. Think of automated forwarding on follow-up and the automated registration of which care provider is attending to the patient and why.

The experience gained in the workflow platform can inspire individual organizations and automate their internal processes, too. This frees up more capacity for direct care interaction, leveraging the investments in the TEC platform.

The workflow functionality of the TEC platform will empower healthcare professionals to make their own OODA loops designed with **Journey Interaction Mapping** (**JIM**) and automate the processes and protocols in incremental steps until autonomy is reached.

For integrated care, all medical data is required to make the integral care plan, which means building the blue line over the systems of medical records, as every integral care plan is based on the automated retrieval of medical data that is available anywhere in the micro-community. As this data is sensitive, the patient has to give consent. Every retrieval action has to be consented to or approved – either for every exchange or waived via a legally accepted mechanism where only a notification is required. This gives maximum flexibility and transparency. The patient keeps track of who is doing what. The privacy policies and rules can be implemented in the IAM functionality of the platform. **Distributed Data Systems** (**DDSs**) and the Solid Pod are suitable technologies to implement the interoperability of the systems of record.

On the systems of engagement side, a life planner that visualizes the overarching integral care plan will stimulate awareness of the importance of health. Systems of intelligence use algorithms to predict and advise possible causes of actions on prevention, early detection, and diagnostics based on all collected data, expanding on the developments of current health-supporting smartwatches.

For directed care, this has been developed even further. The individual's avatar is constantly processing medical, activity, and circumstances data in real time to anticipate the required action in care. On the community side, the care EMC is processing data in real time to predict the required resources to deliver the forecasted care from all individuals in the systems of intelligence.

The systems of intelligence are coupled in such a way that they form an ecosystem to make full use of all available data. The purpose of the **European Health Data Space** (**EHDS**) is to provide a sustainable setup for the use of health data for innovation, research, and other activities. It will result in guardrails and guidelines for the ecosystems we are developing, including enabling systems to empower individuals through increased availability of the proper systems of engagement such as medical devices, systems of record, and systems of intelligence with AI algorithms. The same can be said of Japan's Society 5.0.

But all that processed data has a purpose. It's time to see how to work with that data so that it really serves that purpose.

The quadruple aim for sustainable healthcare

Measuring progress is a challenge in itself. Sustainability is the most challenging and most complex part of the transition. So, how do we measure it with a common understanding?

If we have another look at the value stages, the definitions of costs such as salary and the cost of materials, buildings, and services are well defined. It's only a matter of opinion that defines whether these are high or low. The same applies to team efficiency in processes and the organization's overhead of staff departments such as HR, finance, and IT.

The costs of care provisioning have to be aligned with the reimbursement.

But what about the value of health, lifestyle, and participation in relation to the changing costs because of digitalization and integration?

First, we will take a closer look at three different approaches to handling this topic. They include Triple Aim from IHI, **Value-Based Health Care** (**VBHC**) with **Time-Driven Activity-Based Costing** (**TDABC**), and John Hopkins **Adjusted Clinical Group**® (**ACG**®).

IHI has made a framework in which to measure three qualities: patient experience, population health, and cost per capita. They are widely used all over the world. However, this can only be as accurate as the data allows. Common concerns are that the granularity of the data level is too coarse, is not current, and that it takes a lot of effort to get and aggregate the data. The TEC platform will have to address these concerns as it has to automate the data collection, aggregation, and processing.

In light of personnel shortage, we add job satisfaction as a quality attribute, making a quadruple aim. Otherwise, there is no personnel to go for the triple aim anyway.

Another framework that we mentioned earlier is VBHC. It has six main themes and can be applied to TiSH as follows:

1. Organizing into integrated practice units, such as our micro-enterprise TEC teams

2. Measuring the outcomes and costs for every patient, per TiSH tread

3. Moving to bundled payments for care cycles, as per our value stage

4. Integrating care delivery across separate facilities, applying un- and re-bundling

5. Expanding excellent services across geography, via the learning community

6. Building an enabling IT platform, our TEC platform

The VBHC formula to calculate the value is *Value = Outcomes that matter to patients / Cost per patient.*

Here, the outcomes must be defined very well and registered to make sense. Experiences are very personal. Each community will have to choose their instruments and agree on them. This will take time and can become more elaborate with the values outside healthcare in the higher treads of TiSH.

One tricky part is understanding how to measure and monetize the outcome and how to address the time delay between making the costs and manifesting the outcomes. Investments in prevention will lead to lower care costs somewhere in the future.

On the side of costs, things are somewhat easier. The TDABC approach is an extension of VBHC. For each medical condition, the care delivery value chain is defined, and all of the key activities performed within the entire care cycle are identified. The required direct and indirect resources are mapped per step including the costs per activity and the needed capacity. The sum of all activities is used to calculate the costs.

This approach fits well with the micro-enterprises and activities supported with workflows. In fact, this creates a digital twin of the operations in the set of workflows, which can be used to allocate and calculate costs in near real time. The TEC platform has to enable the data collection for these steps. It's clear that with the increased complexity of the community, it becomes more difficult to get the right data in a timely and automated way. Also, here, maturity has to grow in the community, which will take time.

Then, there is the method of John Hopkins ACG® at the level of the community itself. This population management approach collects data on the health and circumstances of people in the community. This data is assessed in clinical groups and classified in terms of risks (stratified) to care needs. The risk factors, social determinants, and health are translated into what health interventions need to be implemented. The monitoring and evaluation of these outcomes are key to understanding the effects and improving the approach.

Again, the monitoring of outcomes is key to a successful application. Putting the triple aim, VBHC, TDABC, and ACG®, and perhaps other models together to good use will require another topic in terms of maturity. Here, the challenge is to select properly registered data (quality data) using statistical analysis and train AI algorithms to get an accurate digital twin of the community.

The outcomes have to be defined within the community to be able to make decisions on how many resources to allocate to healthcare.

Start on the case management tread by sharing the available financial data to learn from each other and grow with the availability of better data.

With stepped care and the supporting workflows, TDABC can be applied and, along with integrated care, outcomes can be put into the value equation, too.

We place ACG® or another type of population management on the highest tread of TiSH. Fostering population management is a good sign that the transformation has succeeded.

If we go back to our example care provider, the advice for their transformation program zones is to do the following:

- Deploy the sharing of financial data with the other care providers in the community
- Pilot the collection of activity-based costs on one type of stepped-care intervention
- Get involved in a proof of concept or prototype on outcome recording
- Attend a workshop or meeting on population management in the community or initiate this when aspiring for a leading role in the community

This gives a clear road ahead along with expectations for the transformation based on the possibilities of digitization structured with TiSH and JIM. Next, we will take a look at how DevOps4Care can facilitate this road.

Empowering transformation teams

Who is doing the architecting? What is preferable to the TEC teams themselves is to be coached by engineers and consultants and empowered by DevOps4Care. DevOps is about involving all stakeholders. DevOps4Care is for care as the main stakeholder using DevOps to design quick and flexible solutions, becoming even faster and more responsive to the needs of care. This requires automation and a standardized approach to applying DevOps. In IT, we use methodologies such as **Test-Driven Development (TDD)** and **Site Reliability Engineering (SRE)**. Although both methodologies focus on the development of software, we can use these principles in DevOps4Care, too.

In TDD, first, we define the test based on the requirements. Next, the tests are run. This will lead to failures since not every feature has been included yet. The initial tests are meant to fail: this will provide the data to build the product to the exact specifications and fix all the bugs during the iterative process. Tests are rerun every time the product has been improved, up until the point where all tests complete successfully.

SRE mainly focuses on making things easier by automation. Again, it's focusing on software development, but the overarching principle can be used. That principle is about eliminating toil. If a new service or product has been launched, but it causes an increase in the workload for anyone who has to work with the product, it's referred back to the architecting team with the assignment to improve it. This is constantly repeated, up until the product actually does make things easier and the workload is decreased.

The type of DevOps automation that we need has to reduce human assistance to process the 4Care feedback loops so that iterative updates can be deployed faster to applications in production.

The ultimate challenge in the transformation is to automate in such a way that "telling is coding" because automation resources are scarce. It would inhibit the transformation from the lowest ecocycle in the panarchy.

The models utilizing **Model-Based Systems Engineering (MBSE)** and building proper digital twins have to be developed for that. This will be one of the key success factors for the transformation, addressing the key issues during the whole transformation, including panarchy factors, and how and why micro-communities are getting involved.

The processes described in *Chapter 5, Leveraging TiSH as Toolkit for Common Understanding*, with our MoM TiSH as the model of models, CAFCR-REQS, and QFD, are to be automated. Think of capturing the voice of the customer and helping with AI such as DALL.E in an interactive exploration session: new solutions become available by going back and forth between the stories and solutions with SRE. QFD rules are automated to comply with the guardrails, guidelines, and deployment to the decomposition of functions as part of the CAFCR process.

Maturity-driven development is one way to develop the automated and, maybe one day, autonomous DevOps process. It uses Moore's zoning to realize short feedback loops, maybe even on a daily basis, based on a common understanding of the technology with respect to healthcare so that trust is built in the minds and hands of healthcare professionals and, of course, for the health experience of every individual. With this automated DevOps4Care mechanism, we become empowered, allowing us to achieve great things. In the final section of this chapter, let's take a look at the possibilities.

In the next and final chapter, we will land with our feet on the *terra firma* of today again and explore real-world stories. We will see what we can learn from the reflection of real cases using the mental models and the reasonings behind how to use OODA.

Summary

In this chapter, we learned how to bring it all together to take action in the transformation using actionable steps: the shared mental models of TiSH and JIM. We learned how to put these models into action, taking two different approaches to healthcare into consideration. The first approach is the fixing of a health issue, and the second one focuses on alternative solutions that lead to a different lifestyle and health condition.

We learned how TEC teams fulfill a key role in the transformation by architecting, designing, and implementing solutions. They form the bridge between all relevant stakeholders in the transformation process: connecting technology with care and other disciplines such as resource management and connecting various teams and organizations as part of micro-communities. However, the central stakeholder in these communities is always the patient. Finally, we learned in what order transformation steps must be taken to be successful. One important lesson here is to start small and then expand.

There is one last thing to do to conclude this book and that is to practice and hear some stories from the field. In the final chapter, we will learn from the experiences of organizations transforming into sustainable healthcare.

Further reading

Enterprise DevOps for Architects, by Jeroen Mulder, Packt Publishing, 2021

Executing the Transformation

MoM TiSH is proud. Transformation is taking shape. Time to reflect.

This chapter forms the rebar (reinforcing bar) of this book. It fills the last gap in this book and arches over the disciplines involved. By the end of this book, you will be able to reason with and explore architectures together with care professionals, systems engineers, and community builders for new human-centered healthcare. We will include examples from Buurtzorg (International), Nearklinikken (DK), INCA (SUR), and TechnoServe (PER) to discover how these new models can be used to understand their stories.

Finally, we will provide you with an invitation to join the digital transformation of healthcare so that we can shape the future together, regardless of whatever discipline you are in. Strengthening the global community by contributing to the body of knowledge and growing this community to enable healthy lifestyles for prosperous participation in society was the sole purpose of writing this book.

In this chapter, we will cover the following topics:

- Applying OODA to transformation – an exercise
- Recognizing TiSH and DevOps4Care in actual transformations
- Mitigating risks and avoiding pitfalls
- Real-life practices – stories from transformers
- Defining the next steps – building transformative resources

Applying OODA to transformation – an exercise

We ended the previous chapter with our example of a care provider deciding to set up a transformation program. Just launching another project does not solve their experienced dilemmas. This urgency calls for a transformation. We learned how to do that by setting up a task force with the appropriate disciplines, including systems engineers and community builders, along with the care workers.

The main task is to create a common understanding between the disciplines. A common understanding can be created with shared mental models. One is that transformation is done tread by tread along the TiSH staircase and its building blocks. The other is a patient-obsessive approach. We must make sure that the moments of truth in the interactions within the patient's ecosystem are the key activities, which we learned to define with the **Journey Interaction Matrix (JIM)**.

In *Chapter 7, Creating New Platforms with OODA*, we introduced the OODA loop as our principal building block for activities for the shared mental model to bridge or overarch the disciplines of technology, enablers, and care. How does this activity building block relate to the other building blocks?

To lock the building blocks in place for each tread, we need rebar, like the connecting rods used in concrete to make it stronger. This rebar combines the building blocks to form stable treads that can carry the full weight of the provisioning of care, health, lifestyle, and outlook on participation. This weight is formed by the total number of OODA activities.

Hierarchical or tiered OODA loops

While using JIM in *Chapter 8, Learning How Interaction Works in Technology-Enabled Care Teams*, we learned how to define the interactions into a closed OODA loop for each objective. More objectives mean more OODA loops that can influence each other. Think of the medication example added with another objective, wound control, which could be conducted with an ambulant nurse using a smart glass for the tele-expertise of a doctor. Another objective could be cognitive abilities with its own OODA loop of activities. These are all medical health objectives. The municipality could have an objective on lifestyle such as self-reliance in shopping activities. The patient self has the objective to be independent again.

What is the hierarchical relationship between OODA loops in our context? We can use the 4C's of communication, coordination, control, and command for this. This can be seen in the following diagram:

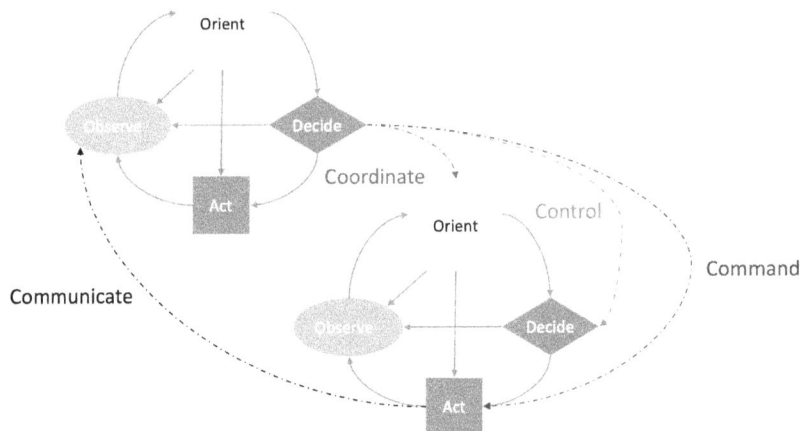

Figure 12.1 – OODA loop relationships

Next to the seven internal relationships between the OODA activities (non-dotted lines), we distinguish four possible external relations with other OODA loops:

- **Communication**: First, communication in a care network is always established. All are communicating what their actions are or have been for others involved in the care network. The teams involved are aware of each other. This is what is needed in case management.

  The other relationships are when one loop needs the other loop to do something. This can be under the discretion of the receiving loop, a joint decision with the other loop, or requires direct action.

  Typically, this results in a hierarchical or tiered situation. From the higher tier to the lower tier, the receiving lower tier has three ways to (re)act.

- **Coordination**: The ability to orient on the decision of the upper tier and decide for themselves. Whatever action is taken is communicated back to the upper tier.

- **Control**: Joint decision-making of both tiers on which action to take.

- **Command**: Execute the action, as decided by the higher tier.

With that, we have defined the different tiers – provisioning, health, lifestyle, and participation. Now, let's see how these relate to the OODA loop and 4C's relationship:

- In case management in ad hoc networks, the providing teams have no hierarchical relationship. There is only the care provisioning tier. However, to be aware of each other in the care network, you must communicate with everyone else involved in the care network. Protocols have to be in place for this – protocols implemented in tools. The team members are trained and skilled to use these tools.

- For stepped care, there are two tiers: the health tier and the care provisioning tier. The relationship between the health tier and care provisioning tier is coordination, where the health tier decided to inform the provisioning tier to consider actions. They have joint responsibility at the health tier. Systems are in place to monitor the health and coordinate the different care provisioning for diagnostics in orientation activities.

- Integrated care has three tiers –lifestyle, health, and provisioning. Joint decision-making is used to control which treatment or intervention is required, and this is done between the lifestyle and health tiers. Here, early detection systems are used to discover possible health issues or lifestyle problems.

- Directed care has four tiers – participation, lifestyle, health, and provisioning. Here, the outlook on participation (or lack of it) leads to action on lifestyle or lower tiers. Here, the person commands the action based on a decision. The person is supported with systems to make such decisions, not only in clear or acute situations with health issues but also to prevent health issues through an adapted lifestyle.

Adding tiers makes the decision-making process more complex, and the subsequent information requirements. However, this also makes the **health experience (HeX)** omniversal, as we depicted in the hexagon that was introduced in the first two chapters of this book.

Next, we are going to look at two examples to make this concrete – one for integrated care and one for directed care.

The following diagram shows the process for integrated care:

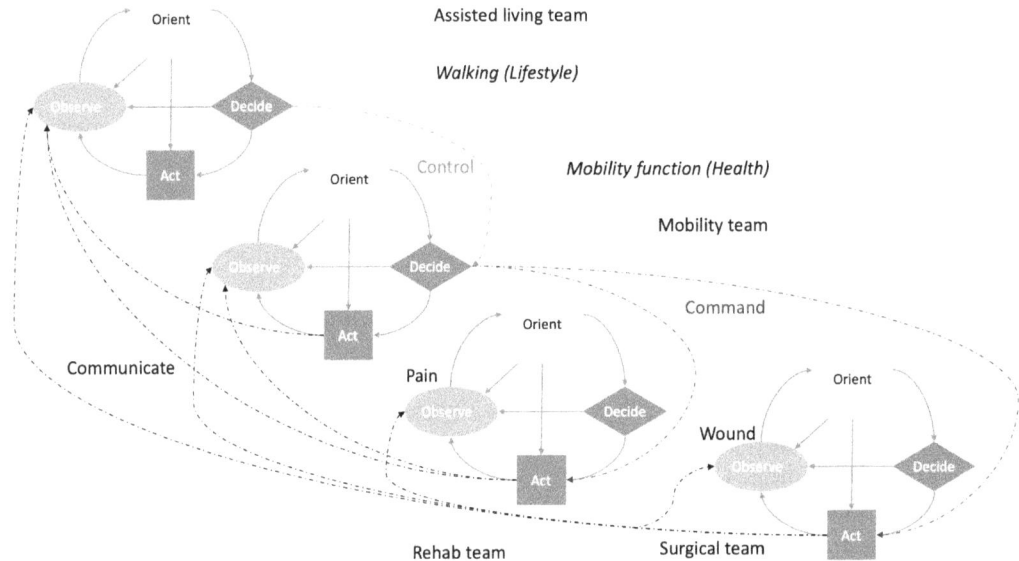

Figure 12.2 – Lifestyle, health, and interventions in integrated care

In this example, the assisted living team is coordinating with the patient on housekeeping support during the rehabilitation period. This assistance compensates for not being able to participate due to the immobility caused by a hip replacement. Being able to walk again is the main wish of the patient.

A joint decision between the patient and assisted living team is made in this integrated care to focus on mobility first and wait for cognitive treatment. This decision controls (the dotted line) the priority of the mobility team. The team is using the patient's main wish in their decision-making.

Two teams are doing the actual interventions under command (the dotted line) of the mobility team, the rehab team for the exercises and pain medication, and the surgical team to monitor the wound caused by the hip replacement. The cognitive team is not shown but they were involved in the joint decision-making and observe the results without any action.

For this, the platform has a mobility dashboard for everyone to see and use for the decision and define workflows to support integrated care.

These workflows adhere to the guidelines on mobility care, as agreed to due to acknowledged cooperation. In this case, the value the cooperation delivers is mobility. Both social and medical teams are involved.

The following diagram is for directed care:

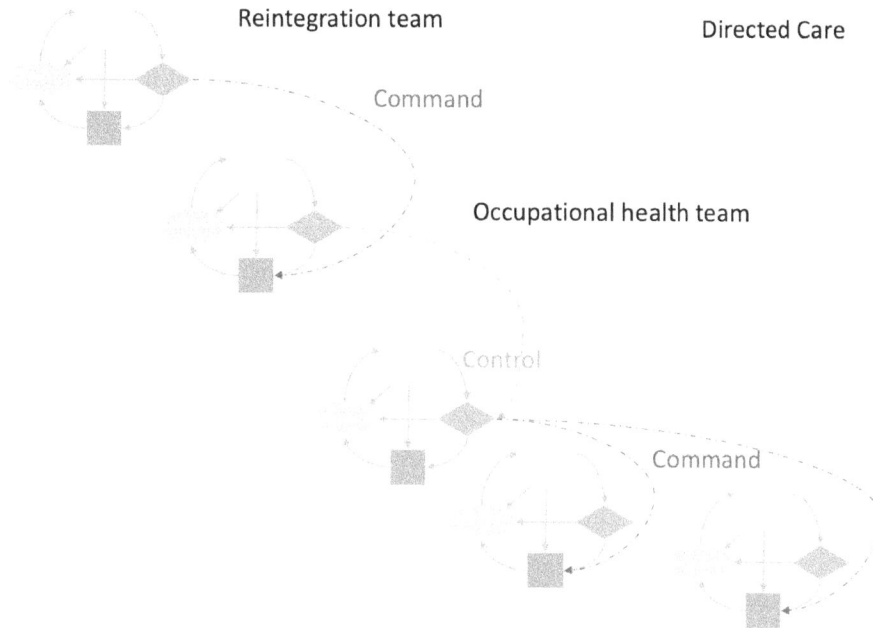

Figure 12.3 – Participation, lifestyle, health, and interventions in directed care

An example of directed care is from the perspective of participating in work. Here, orders are issued (commanded) from the reintegration team to the occupational health team. The occupational health team operates itself as integrated care and controls the different types of interventions to reintegrate workers. This can also be interventions in the working environment, preventative individual behavior, and early detection of injuries.

These small examples demonstrated how to model the activities and information requirements for them in comprehensive interaction maps. Information that flows in real or near-real time through workflows supports the activities in the OODA loops.

The question is, can you model these information requirements? First, you must make a Journey Interaction Map that contains several interrelated OODA loops of the care you are involved in. Secondly, you must translate each step into the necessary information requirements.

Information requirements must be provided to the developers of the enabling entities, as discussed in *Chapter 9, Working with Complex (System of) Systems*.

This brings us back to the other building blocks. Let's see how the rebar weaving we presented here can be applied to the transformation.

Recognizing TiSH and DevOps4Care in actual transformations

Now that we've introduced the 4C and OODA loop relationships, including the hierarchical tiers of decision-making, we can complete the building blocks of the TiSH staircase, starting from the upper tier of participation.

In terms of the ICF model, the major life areas are work, education or community, and social and civic life activities. The outlook on this participation will result in decisions on the lifestyle tier surrounding activities such as mobility, learning, and general tasks within the environmental factors. Think of working conditions – the health tier is about the body's functions and structures in terms of the physical, mental, and intellectual functioning of people.

The following diagram shows the entire model with all the building blocks:

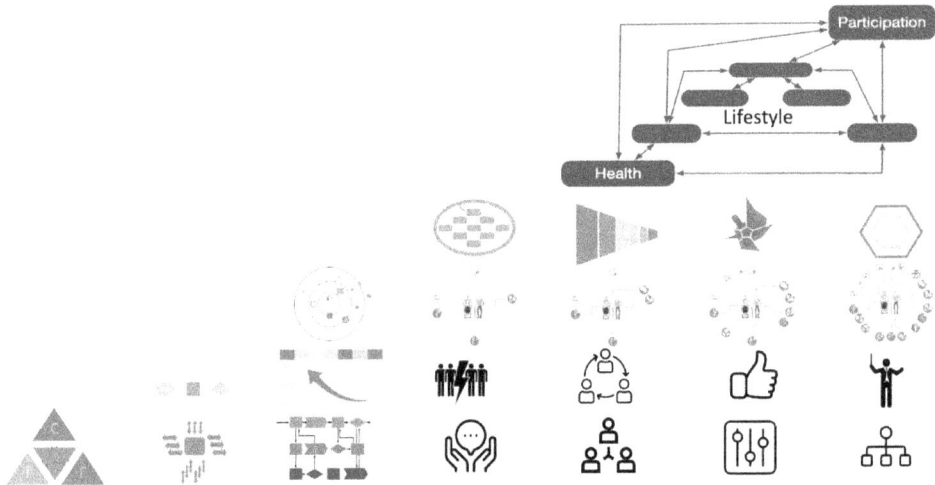

Figure 12.4 – TiSH staircase with all its building blocks

Depending on which tier will take responsibility, the network tier has four types, from case management in ad hoc networks to directed care. Each has more demanding types of decision-making.

The organization tier uses the Rendanheyi principles of rebundling teams within the care networks around the person with enough capacity. This tier also defines the enabling platform. This tier is the key tier in the transformation since it knows that the complexity of the enabling platform increases with each tread.

The teams tier is about preparing capable teams to work on OODA activities and OODA loops for health journeys with ever-increasing complexity, helping them grow their capabilities and apply these to the decisions they take in the care networks.

Finally, the foundational personal tier focuses on activities and their interactions while following workflows and growing people's skills so that they can work in the communication, coordination, control, and command structures.

To apply this in DevOps4Care, we can focus on decision-making expressed as part of the activities in the OODA loops. We will create a shared mental model with a comprehensive interaction map to help with this:

- Care professionals such as clinicians, nurses, and practitioners in medical terms act as the 4Care component.

- Technicians who derive the requirements for the components and systems of the platform act as the Dev component.

- Enablers who can translate the understanding into entities for operations or Ops.

With this complete model, we can conclude that we learned to reason about the interrelated aspects of transformation and to explore stories in a structured (modeled) narrative with other disciplines.

With that, we have given you the scaffolding, building blocks, and rebar weaving to make your transformation concrete. However, there will always be risks.

Mitigating risks and avoiding pitfalls

Although we could write entire books on risks, we will address them here at a principles level. Risks are always there and mitigation mechanisms have to be in place.

To avoid pitfalls, we must follow three principles:

- Value inhibition in the panarchy ecocycles, as mentioned in *Chapter 6*, *Applying the Panarchy Principle*

- Leadership

- Learning

We will look at these principles in the next section.

Anticipating inhibitions

We recall here the deceleration forces in *Figure 6. 5* of not aligned values in the ecocycle above your own ecocycle. The decision-makers involved in the ecocycle who are determining the investments must be involved at a very early stage. They must all look for ways to solve their dilemmas. A sense of urgency must exist.

Be sure not to skip a tier or ecocycle of the panarchy. Brilliant ideas in a team using new technologies such as VR in metaverses are indeed ideas. Proof of concepts and pilots are needed to build evidence that a solution can solve a problem worth investing in. Again, you must involve decision-makers as early as possible. Make sure that you understand each other. This goes for both decision-makers in the medical field and finances.

Taking your time with the transformation is the best mitigation. The less understanding there is, the more underestimation of time that's needed. Embrace the complexity by understanding it and make realistic plans for the transformations. This is where leadership comes in.

Leadership

Leadership is something we touch on in the Rendanheyi approach for ecosystem micro-communities, which involves self-organizing, self-governing, and self-motivating micro-enterprises enabled by platforms and united in a common purpose and by common values and a common strategic vision on networked care. We are quick to say that we are not leadership experts but sometimes, an interesting concept comes to our attention that's in line with the Rendanheyi thought leadership.

Recently, a Healthtech scale-up called Luscii published their view on leadership with *"Green ON, the most pleasant and productive way of working."* The two founders, Joris Janssen and Daan Dohmen, teamed up with yet another example from the military, the special forces. See the *Further reading* section for more details on their publication.

They also emphasize the independent way of working of the teams by using roles and taking decisions with what they call a minimum viable group. Trust the ones who know best, the ones who are most informed, and the ones who take responsibility for the situation or event at hand.

Decisions should be made in real time, on the fly, and not in planned meetings that focus on urgent issues. This fits well with OODA's focus on the mission objectives and quick loop iterations to test whether something works and if not, learn from it quickly.

This brings us to learning.

Learn

Learn and learn quickly – not only from yourself but from others as well. Again, a common understanding is key here.

From this, we can conclude that the biggest pitfall is not making enough time and effort to embrace the complexity and oversimplify the transformation.

Real-life practices – stories from transformers

In this section, we will look at the terra firma of today once more and explore real-world stories. We will see what we can learn from reflecting on real cases using various mental models and the reasoning behind them.

Gerben Krehwinkel, Treant Group, The Netherlands

Gerben Krehwinkel is the IT director of the Dutch Treant group. This group operates hospitals and care homes in the northern part of the Netherlands. One crucial observation that Gerben made was that IT and the medical staff of the group didn't speak the same language – they came from different planets. *"We provided iPads for patient monitoring to nurses, but they were all sent back to IT. It didn't work. But, no one explained exactly what it was that didn't work. Hence, the only thing that IT did was reinstall the iPads and return them to the staff. If you don't know what problem you're fixing, you're not fixing anything at all. The real problem was that the nurses didn't know what to do with the iPads."*

The IT landscape was fragmented and not standardized, which in itself acts as an inhibition to move forward and think of innovations. That was the start of an innovation program that Gerben designed with his team. It consisted of five pillars: basic infrastructure, home automation, innovation platform, eHealth, and the care professional, which is the most important pillar of all.

The basic infrastructure is about having good Wi-Fi connections in all buildings, for instance. But it also specifies the standardization of the workplaces and security controls. These should be the same in all hospitals and homes of the group. It's the foundation for everything else. Treant learned a lot from assessing home automation in various buildings. *"That was old technology,"* says Krehwinkel. *"Think of the social alarm button that a patient needs to press to call a nurse. But before we could install new technology, we needed to upgrade and standardize the infrastructure."*

The third and central pillar is the innovation platform. This is not about technology in the first place, but about people. *"In this pillar, we talk with care professionals about innovation. Clinicians, nurses, and patients are all represented on this platform. The platform also maintains intensive contact with the outside world: we can't do everything by ourselves, and besides, there's no reason to reinvent the wheel. We often discover that something has already been done before, something that we can reuse."*

This cumulates in the fourth pillar: eHealth. "*This is the pillar where we try things. The smart glass is a good example. We started with a small pilot, with only two pairs of glasses. Next, we implemented it for wound care, so that a clinician could remotely view what the nurse would see when a patient's wound was treated. Now, we have these glasses in all our locations. We follow the same roadmap for the implementation of hip airbags for patients that are unstable and tend to fall frequently, with the risk of breaking their hip, and the voice-controlled care app that our staff uses to update patient files. In the innovation platform, we decide if something adds value, then we test it extensively, run pilots, and eventually scale up. Everything that we introduced using this path has been successfully implemented.*"

The fifth pillar is crucial in this process: the care professional. This is the pillar where staff members are trained. "*The creative process that drives innovation must come from the people who have to deal with patients daily: our medical staff. A certain technology might be wonderful, but there's always one question that must be answered. How does it add value to the care of our patients? To be able to assess the possibilities and try things, you need to have professionals in the innovation teams. This means that you must train people and take them with you on that journey.*"

Treant is still at the beginning, says Krehwinkel. "*The adoption curve takes a long time. You need to be aware of that: you can't force things top-down. An example: in one of the homes where we treat Alzheimer's patients, we introduced an app that was connected to a sensor, showing if patients were lying in their bed at night, not wandering around. The nurse could track the patients using that app. The first thing we noticed was that the nurses would prefer to check the patients themselves; they didn't trust the image in the app. That's a matter of adoption and that takes time.*"

In terms of TiSH, we put Treant on tread two. They are building capable teams to transform healthcare. Rebundling is on the way with the example of the smart glass for wound control. So, tread three is in sight. Our curiosity is in how quickly Treant will be on the treads of networked care. Having a lot of history and established culture will probably lead to some *not letting go* inhibitions. On the other hand, agreements with other care providers have already been signed to jointly develop networked care.

Dr. Javier Asin, Surinam

In *Chapter 1, Understanding (the Need for) Transformation*, we introduced integrated care and stepped care while using the spider web models that have been developed by Dr. Javier Asin.

"*We noticed that there was a problem with patients with multiple chronic diseases. The diseases were all treated with different programs that were not interconnected nor integrated,*" explains Asin. "*The problem starts with the fact that every treatment has its own standards and protocols. Take a patient with diabetes as an example. Not every form of diabetes is like the others. The protocol states how diabetes must be treated, but it doesn't tell us how diabetes must be treated when the patient also suffers from COPD.*" That's where Asin started developing the INCA program: Integrated Care.

The idea is simple: treatment is not described per disease, but per problem. "*A lot of patients have multiple issues impacting their health: too much weight, they might be smoking, or they might have mental issues. This all impacts the effect of the treatment. Hence, it must be taken into consideration, specifically for that patient. A standard program to treat disease will not result in the desired effect. It also means that caregivers have to collaborate in creating an individual program for that patient. They have to step outside of their standards and protocols and focus on what that patient needs.*"

This results in an individual plan. The next challenge is to motivate the patient. "*A doctor focuses on clinical values and decides on a treatment based on those values. To a patient, these values are likely nothing more than just some numbers – a score. They don't reflect the actual feeling of the patient. That's why we developed the spider web: it makes things clear and visible. The more a problem gets to the outside of the web, the bigger the problem. It tells the patient exactly what they need to work on. Then, it's up to the patient to start the work: together with their doctor, they decide where to start. That might be losing weight or quitting smoking, instead of starting the immediate treatment of a specific disease. The goal is that in the end, the patient feels better and can take part in society again. It doesn't necessarily mean that a disease must be cured as a priority. We must understand what the patient wants and then who does what and when in terms of treatment.*"

In the latest versions of the spider web, socio-economic issues have been added since they can heavily influence the well-being of a patient. Think of issues with income, work, or issues concerning loneliness, with the latter becoming a growing problem among elderly patients.

The program was tested successfully in clinics in Surinam, but unfortunately, it was recently stopped because of governmental decisions, emphasizing the need to have all stakeholders in healthcare fully on board.

This is an example of tread six of integrated care targeting lifestyle problems. However, it was a pilot and the move to full deployment was inhibited at the society ecocycle level. The value of better lifestyles is not leading to policy changes. The next step would be to form a governing body such as the Cooperation Committee, as described in *Table 9.5*.

The same inhibition is also true for the Nearklinikken in Denmark. Although studies show a benefit of the stepped care approach with ECM, the financing after the project funding is not yet clear.

Vingtoft says that what they need is a health bank, where something such as a shared savings model can make sure that their approach has sustainable value for everyone.

And not only small initiatives encounter this inhibition point. At the time of writing, Amazon Care announced that it will stop with its endeavor because the approach was not deemed sustainable. Instead, they will pursue the acquisition of One Medical, which can be described as a case management subscription or, in their words, something "*to help navigate the healthcare maze.*" This is tread four in terms of TiSH, but with a clear objective that focuses on health and lifestyle and with the subscription issued as an employee benefit coupled with participation as value for the employers. This bridges the value stages between tread four, reimbursement value, and tread seven, economic value, which is more sustainable.

Another sustainable success is Buurtzorg. Let's take a look.

Geert Quint

Geert Quint was involved in organizing the IT for Buurtzorg, the organization that Jos de Blok founded as an alternative to the more traditional institutions that delivered care to the homes of patients. *"The issue was that we had the technology available to improve the work of caregivers, but the caregivers themselves were not prepared to work with that technology,"* says Quint.

The principle idea from the start was to give professionals the software that they needed, in a **Software-as-a-Service** (**SaaS**) model. That software, developed by Ecare, was designed in such a way that it provided freedom in usage, enabling professionals to make choices and decisions for themselves, not fully directed by company rules or standards. *"That's the model of Buurtzorg: self-management; letting go of procedures that are simply too rigid. These procedures might not always fit the needs of a patient."*

Quint has seen a lot of changes since Buurtzorg started and the software that Ecare developed. Technology has played an important role in that. *"The challenge is always the funding: who's paying for the innovation? Take the medicine dispensers that pharmacies have today. It was a perfect solution to get patients to use the right doses, preventing waste of medicines. Once the insurance companies saw the added value of this, the solution was implemented at scale."*

The Ecare software for Buurtzorg was another good example. It was easy to use for the care professionals. *"It was easy to use for updating patient files and easy to communicate with others. Updating files took just a couple of minutes. It was scaled to a lot of teams, but they all used a shared platform, built on public Azure and Google clouds. The best part was that the founder, Jos, also used the platform to publish his blogs. Staff could immediately provide feedback, which was extremely valuable in further shaping the organization. Feedback was processed directly in new releases. We could do several releases per day."*

That's key in developing and implementing solutions in healthcare. *"First, you have to keep it very simple, something that is easy to scale. Secondly, you need collaboration in the entire chain. All stakeholders must be involved. Technology requires investments. This will only be done when stakeholders see the value of the investments."*

We do not have to add much here. What's key is that the nurses, who are looking after the patients, are capable of making decisions, providing that they have up-to-date information and can inform each other quickly, and are not distracted by the enabling systems. With this, they can also play their role in any type of networked care. This is at the core of Buurtzorg's international success.

Pamela Girano

Pamela Girano is the country director of TechnoServe, a **Non-Governmental Organization** (**NGO**) that helps people lift themselves out of poverty by harnessing the power of the private sector. We asked Pamela what role healthcare plays in their efforts. Although not directly involved in healthcare, she knows that the areas they work for are often the areas where access to healthcare is difficult.

For example, in Peru, thousands of farmers are helped to grow crops economically. However, these farmers and their communities, 77% of the time, lack communication network coverage. So, when someone is left injured during farming or due to an illness, farming is jeopardized.

One example she told was that a farmer broke their leg on their farmland with no way to ask for help. Only by crawling to the road and the luck of someone passing by were they able to get some help in a nearby village. After this, it took a few weeks for the farmer to heal and work the land again. Access to healthcare would improve participation in the local community.

The inhibition to getting better healthcare is connectivity. But why should a community or business invest in such a service? To see if such a service could provide other forms of value that a community could decide to invest in. For example, the same communication could give access to crop forecasting based on satellite images.

Here, a potential economic value can be the driver too. The shared platform could start with a community satellite dish such as Starlink to use for eConsults with doctors in cities and to get local nurses trained. The community village elders could act as the governance to manage these collective steps. Again, the expertise of TechnoServe could help make the community aware of these possibilities.

The message here is that transforming something from almost nothing can bring great leaps forward when worldwide accessible resources are used, starting with the participation view rather than transforming from a traditional care provisioning view.

Defining the next steps – building transformative resources

Organizing **Transformation Events** in practice needs preparation. Using the iceberg model of systems thinking depicted as follows, one has to learn the use of models as presented in TiSH; internalize them into **Mental models**; and explore them jointly, becoming **Shared Mental models**; then apply these in **Community Structures** like **Ecosystem Micro Enterprises** and plan **Patterns of Chance** using OODA.

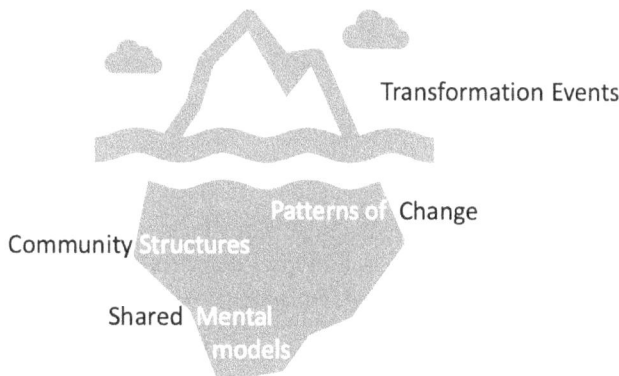

Figure 12.5 – Transformation Iceberg

With this sequence in mind, the next step is to get access to the required skills of systems engineering and community builders. It's here that we invite anyone with experience in these fields but who is not yet involved in healthcare to connect to the healthcare transformation community. Increasing their involvement will increase the speed of healthcare transformation.

Then, they must join forces in developing automated DevOps. Making the tools to take the narrative from care workers to code for improved platforms will also increase the speed of healthcare transformation.

With these two main steps, we are building transformative resources with enough capacity and not getting stuck in the trap of good ideas but no execution power.

We hope you join us and explore the future.

Exploring the future of technology

Finally, let's talk about the future. Using the DevOps4Care mechanism, the adoption of new technologies becomes pull-based and the advances in technology can be transformed into value quicker. Each day, devices become more powerful and smaller. Computing is an incredible shrinking machine that's becoming more and more available in any point of care environment. To anticipate what is possible over the coming years, we can consider the evolution of this incredible shrinking machine. It's Moore's law put into the form factor of computing devices.

The form factor size has been roughly developed as follows:

- Ca. 1945 – Building size (ENIAC)
- Ca. 1960 – Cabinet size (PDP-1 minicomputer)
- Ca. 1975 – Box size (PET, Altair, and other personal or microcomputers)
- Ca. 1990 – Book size (laptops)
- Ca. 2005 – Palm-size (smartphones)
- Ca. 2020 – Wearable (smartwatch, smart glasses, and VR sets)

With some speculation, the form factors can shrink to the following sizes:

- Ca. 2035 – Implantable, such as an ID chip, which is only a few millimeters in size
- Ca. 2050 – Injectable nano-machines

Note that some larger implantables are already in use in the form of pacemakers, glucose pumps, or artificial organs such as an artificial pancreas for type-1 diabetics or even artificial hearts. We are already living in the generation of wearables, and implantables will follow suit.

This has consequences for the guardrails and guidelines, so we have to be ready for this. The research ecosystem micro-communities have to fit in so that the other communities can learn to use and build the supporting solutions at an early stage, becoming **Research & Development (R&D)** Ops4Care.

Ethical issues have to be tackled. What does it mean if information becomes an integral part of the body and person? This should at least be reflected in the facilities for user classes through the ultimate micro-segmentation in the IAM functionality of the TEC platform.

We use reasoning to think things through to explore joint solutions and truly embrace the complexity of the transformation. We use maturity-driven program management for each step on the treads of the TiSH staircase. We apply JIM and apply rebar weaving to the TEC platform with the panarchy and available technology in mind. By doing this relentlessly, we can realize the full potential of Society 5.0 and even possibly evolve into the transhuman era.

Summary

Throughout this book, we drew the plans, formed the teams, and defined a good strategy using TiSH, putting it together into a transformation program. This resulted in an architecture for achieving sustainable healthcare. We addressed some of the most common pitfalls and how to avoid or mitigate these. In this final chapter, we illustrated this transformation with real-life examples, through the stories of people doing the actual transformations.

This chapter was a full recap of everything we have learned, but it focused on how to apply the principles of DevOps. In essence, DevOps is about setting an ambition and then iterating toward that ambition while learning from every step we take. The OODA loops and eco cycles are a perfect way of learning and overcoming inhibitions. Technology plays an important role in transforming healthcare, but it all starts with the patients and the caregivers who need to work with the technology. Throughout this book, we have been emphasizing this. TiSH, JIM, and the principles of Rendanheyi will provide teams with the proper tools for executing the transformation.

We thank you for your interest in the subject of healthcare transformation and the time you took to read this book. We hope that it will prove worthwhile in helping you decide to get involved in healthcare in the first place, use these insights to embrace the complexity in your work to innovate and transform healthcare, or help the healthcare transformation community to further their **Body of Knowledge (BoK)**, such as by creating learning paths to help the community grow and make knowledge more widely available for healthcare worldwide.

Further reading

Green ON, by Joris Janssen, Daan Dohmen, Richard Bergmans, Thomas de Jong, Frank van Drenthe, Green ON publishers, 2022.

Index

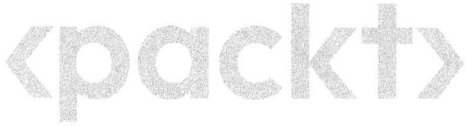

‹packt›

Subscribe to our online digital library for full access to over 7,000 books and videos, as well as industry leading tools to help you plan your personal development and advance your career. For more information, please visit our website.

Why subscribe?

- Spend less time learning and more time coding with practical eBooks and Videos from over 4,000 industry professionals

- Improve your learning with Skill Plans built especially for you

- Get a free eBook or video every month

- Fully searchable for easy access to vital information

- Copy and paste, print, and bookmark content

Did you know that Packt offers eBook versions of every book published, with PDF and ePub files available? You can upgrade to the eBook version at packt.com and as a print book customer, you are entitled to a discount on the eBook copy. Get in touch with us at customercare@packtpub.com for more details.

At www.packt.com, you can also read a collection of free technical articles, sign up for a range of free newsletters, and receive exclusive discounts and offers on Packt books and eBooks.

Other Books You May Enjoy

If you enjoyed this book, you may be interested in these other books by Packt:

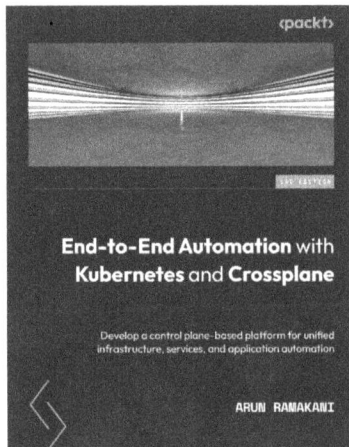

End-to-End Automation with Kubernetes and Crossplane

Arun Ramakani

ISBN: 9781801811545

- Understand the context of Kubernetes-based infrastructure automation
- Get to grips with Crossplane concepts with the help of practical examples
- Extend Crossplane to build a modern infrastructure automation platform
- Use the right configuration management tools in the Kubernetes environment
- Explore patterns to unify application and infrastructure automation
- Discover top engineering practices for infrastructure platform as a product

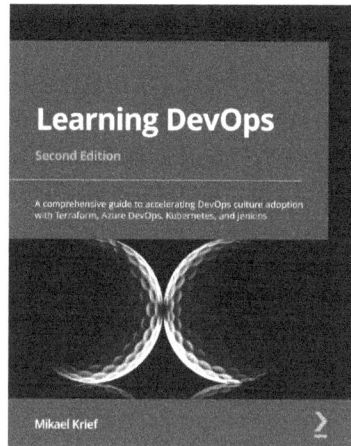

Learning DevOps - Second Edition

Mikael Krief

ISBN: 9781801818964

- Understand the basics of infrastructure as code patterns and practices

- Get an overview of Git command and Git flow

- Install and write Packer, Terraform, and Ansible code for provisioning and configuring cloud infrastructure based on Azure examples

- Use Vagrant to create a local development environment

- Containerize applications with Docker and Kubernetes

- Apply DevSecOps for testing compliance and securing DevOps infrastructure

- Build DevOps CI/CD pipelines with Jenkins, Azure Pipelines, and GitLab CI

- Explore blue-green deployment and DevOps practices for open sources projects

Packt is searching for authors like you

If you're interested in becoming an author for Packt, please visit `authors.packtpub.com` and apply today. We have worked with thousands of developers and tech professionals, just like you, to help them share their insight with the global tech community. You can make a general application, apply for a specific hot topic that we are recruiting an author for, or submit your own idea.

Share your thoughts

Now you've finished *Transforming Healthcare with DevOps*, we'd love to hear your thoughts! Scan the QR code below to go straight to the Amazon review page for this book and share your feedback or leave a review on the site that you purchased it from.

`https://packt.link/r/1801817316`

Your review is important to us and the tech community and will help us make sure we're delivering excellent quality content.

Download a free PDF copy of this book

Thanks for purchasing this book!

Do you like to read on the go but are unable to carry your print books everywhere? Is your eBook purchase not compatible with the device of your choice?

Don't worry, now with every Packt book you get a DRM-free PDF version of that book at no cost.

Read anywhere, any place, on any device. Search, copy, and paste code from your favorite technical books directly into your application.

The perks don't stop there, you can get exclusive access to discounts, newsletters, and great free content in your inbox daily

Follow these simple steps to get the benefits:

1. Scan the QR code or visit the link below

https://packt.link/free-ebook/9781801817318

2. Submit your proof of purchase
3. That's it! We'll send your free PDF and other benefits to your email directly

www.ingramcontent.com/pod-product-compliance
Lightning Source LLC
Chambersburg PA
CBHW061354210326
41598CB00035B/5988